Praise for *Fed* [...]

"In the last couple of decades we have becom[...] will automatically breastfeed their infants; ho[...] has resulted in negative consequences for both [...] [m]other. Nobody denies that human milk is the gold standard fo[...] infants but we have failed to also endorse that well-fed infants should be the gold standard. This well-balanced book is intended to support our mothers, fathers, and all the people involved in the journey of newborn feedings by bringing up the realities of different feeding methods so that parents can make an informed choice. This book will encourage parents and providers to understand that each couple is different and needs to be fully supported to achieve a successful feeding journey."

—Enrique Gomez, MD, MSc, pediatrician and neonatologist

"*Fed Is Best* is a masterfully written book and a profound contribution to making medical complications from insufficient feeding of breastfed babies a 'never-ever event.' It is a must-read for every lactation care provider, pediatrician, and expectant parent."

—Marianne Neifert, MD, FAAP, cofounder of the Academy of Breastfeeding Medicine

"*Fed Is Best* bravely tells the truth: babies thrive on breast milk, formula, or a combination of the two. May everyone who cares about families, science, or public health shout it from the rooftops."

—Joan Wolf, associate professor of women and gender studies at Texas A&M University

"*Fed Is Best*. It seems so straightforward. The most important thing is to make sure your baby is fed. That's the simple premise of this important book that explains how 'breast is best' has led mothers and doctors to prioritize breastfeeding over making sure a baby is eating, with results that have endangered babies' health and even lives. Crucially, the authors don't just stop there. Their practical advice teaches new parents how to recognize the danger signs of underfeeding and what to do about it. And it meets new parents where they are, with chapters on breastfeeding, pumped milk feeding, formula feeding, combination feeding, and bottle feeding with breastmilk or formula. The message is clear. There are many good ways to feed a baby. If you or someone in your life is having a baby, this is the book to buy. It's thoughtful and clear, and it prioritizes a baby's health over ideology and dogma. No matter where you end up on your feeding journey, this book will help parents protect their babies."

—Courtney Jung, professor and George Ignatieff chair in peace and conflict studies at the University of Toronto

FED
IS BEST

The Unintended Harms of the "Breast Is Best" Message and How to Find the Right Approach for You and Your Baby

Christie del Castillo-Hegyi, MD
B. Jody Segrave-Daly, RN, IBCLC RETIRED
with **Lynnette Hafken,** MA, IBCLC

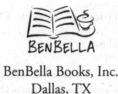

BenBella Books, Inc.
Dallas, TX

BenBella

BenBella Books, Inc.
10440 N. Central Expressway
Suite 800
Dallas, TX 75231
benbellabooks.com
Send feedback to feedback@benbellabooks.com

BenBella is a federally registered trademark.

Printed in the United States of America
10 9 8 7 6 5 4 3 2 1

Library of Congress Control Number: 2023053078
ISBN 9781637744628 (trade paperback)
ISBN 9781637744635 (electronic)

Editing by Leah Wilson
Copyediting by James Fraleigh
Proofreading by Lisa Story and Rebecca Maines
Indexing by Wordco Indexing Services
Text design and composition by PerfecType, Nashville, TN
Cover design by Oceana Garceau
Cover image © iStock / Yoshikitaima
Printed by Lake Book Manufacturing

Dedicated to all families seeking safe and inclusive infant feeding support that allows the whole family to thrive

CONTENTS

IMPORTANT NOTES

The purpose of this book is to provide science-based infant feeding information to the public based on the most current peer-reviewed litera-ture. The authors and the Fed Is Best Foundation used their medical and scientific judgment to select these resources. The contents of this book are provided as an informational resource only and should not be relied upon as medical advice for diagnostic or treatment purposes. The information is not intended for any specific patient, and receipt of this book from a healthcare professional or the Fed Is Best Foundation does not create a client–consultant or patient–clinician/patient–doctor relationship. **There is no substitute for professional diagnosis and treatment.**

Contact your child's physician for information about specific medical conditions and your child's nutritional and medical needs. Never disregard or delay seeking professional medical advice because of something you have read in this book or any other resource.

The Fed Is Best Foundation does not recommend or endorse any spe-cific tests, physicians, products, or procedures. The Foundation also does not accept funds or other donations from any organization or corporation that produces and sells goods and services related to newborn, infant, or toddler feeding, including products and services relating to breastfeeding and formula feeding. All of the authors' portion of the proceeds from this book are going to the Fed Is Best Foundation.

Science-based infant feeding information changes over time, and it is the responsibility of the reader to verify that they are relying on the most up-to-date information to make decisions about infant feeding and management. The information in this book is based on the medical and scientific information available at the time of publication, and that information may evolve and become outdated with time. As a result, it is important to consult with a healthcare professional to ensure that you have the most current information, and to watch for future editions of this book. If you have questions about the information in this book, consult your child's physician.

A NOTE ABOUT INCLUSIVE LANGUAGE

The authors of this book and the Fed Is Best Foundation strive to educate in a manner that is inclusive of people of all races, ethnicities, nationalities, socioeconomic classes, belief systems, family structures, gender identities, and sexual orientations. While the English language is imperfect at representing gender identity, we strive to refer to every member of our audience, which includes cis mothers and fathers, trans mothers and fathers, and non-binary parents, both biological and adoptive. In this book, we alternate among using the terms *mother*, *parent*, *she/her*, and *they/them* to refer to the birthing and/or lactating parent.

CONTENT WARNING

Some of the following information may be shocking or upsetting, as it discusses preventable conditions that cause harm to infants and their families. You may choose to learn the signs of sufficient and insufficient feeding from the tables on pages 77 and 85, then skip ahead to part 2, the instructional portion of the book. Our online resources, like the Fed Is Best Feeding Plan, are available through QR-coded links throughout the book and provide guidance on how to work toward your personal infant-feeding goals while ensuring safe and adequate feeding.

INTRODUCTION

Christie's Story and the Birth of Fed Is Best

As a physician and expectant first-time mother, I had no doubt that I would exclusively breastfeed my first-born child. I read a popular breastfeeding book and attended my hospital's breastfeeding classes to prepare. I had a healthy pregnancy, and my son was born after an uncomplicated vaginal delivery, weighing 8 pounds, 11 ounces. He was placed on my belly and latched on well immediately. He woke up about every three hours and I fed him for twenty to thirty minutes on demand.

We stayed in the hospital for two days, during which time we were visited by a pediatrician and an International Board Certified Lactation Consultant (IBCLC) each day of our stay. The IBCLC noted that my son's latch was perfect. He developed jaundice by the second day, although his levels were unremarkable. He had lost 5 percent of his birth weight and produced the expected number of wet and dirty diapers upon discharge at forty-eight hours. Our first two days were exactly as the breastfeeding books described. Before discharge, the IBCLC told me that he would be hungry and to just keep putting him to the breast and he would get enough colostrum, the first milk that mothers produce after birth.

We went home, and as predicted, he was hungry. So, I fed him longer and longer into the night. He would cry after latching on and I would

1

put him back on the breast. He did not sleep. My husband and I were baffled by how demanding it was. After a long night of breastfeeding, we saw our pediatrician the next morning. We were told our son had now lost 1 pound, 3 ounces, which we weren't informed represented 15 percent of his birth weight. He was jaundiced, but his bilirubin level (the blood test for jaundice) was not checked. Perhaps to keep from discouraging me, our pediatrician told us we could either supplement or keep breastfeeding frequently and wait for my milk to come in on day four or five. We decided to try one more day of breastfeeding without supplementation, and I fed near-continuously.

By his fourth day of life, we saw another IBCLC, who weighed him before and after nursing and discovered he had gotten absolutely no milk through breastfeeding. When I expressed and pumped, not a drop of milk came out.

I shook with fatigue and terror. I imagined the four days of life-endangering torture I had put my child through. We fed him formula from the sample our pediatrician gave us once we returned home, and he finally fell asleep. When my husband went to get him from his nap three hours later, he was unresponsive.

As an emergency physician, I recognized he was hypoglycemic—his blood sugar was too low. I quickly prepared a bottle of formula, which my husband squeezed into his mouth. He swallowed it and became more alert. But then he immediately started seizing. We rushed him to the emergency room and found that he had a barely normal glucose level, severe jaundice (commonly known as breastfeeding jaundice), and a severe form of dehydration called hypernatremia. I had only seen hypernatremia that severe in comatose patients with dementia who had not drunk water in days. Having done newborn brain injury research in college, I realized he had starved—and that it had profoundly injured his brain.

At that moment, I wondered why this had happened, when the books assured me that not producing enough breast milk was rare. If it was so rare, why were my colleagues acting as if this was a routine occurrence? As I was explaining to the neonatologist why this had happened, I began to say that it was because my milk had not come in but couldn't finish the sentence out of shame. She guessed the end. Then she assured me, "Your son will be fine." Didn't she see that his laboratory data clearly indicated that he had sustained brain injury and that my previously perfectly healthy newborn would potentially be disabled for the rest of his life? Were they hiding it from me, or did they not know? What would the future consequences of his brain injury be, and why had I not heard of this kind of thing happening before?

If this had happened to two physicians taking home their first-born child, it had to be happening to an unimaginable number of new parents who weren't medical professionals. I remembered breastfeeding jaundice being mentioned briefly during medical school, but no one had ever described what it really meant: that a baby could spend days starving at the breast, even to the point of brain injury or death. In a world where a million cribs are recalled if one baby dies, why had no one warned me that this apparently common, life-threatening, and potentially disabling event could happen to my child—and that I could have prevented it with formula?

Exclusive breastfeeding from birth to six months is recommended by the World Health Organization (WHO), UNICEF, the Centers for Disease Control and Prevention (CDC), and the American Academy of Pediatrics (AAP), among others. It means giving only breast milk, preferably through direct nursing, with no additional food, water, or formula from birth to six months, with rare medical exceptions.[1] The most prominent advice I had read and learned from breastfeeding classes and books was to avoid formula to prevent breastfeeding failure and long-term health problems for my child. Not *once* was I informed of the even worse health consequences of not feeding my child enough while following these guidelines. I lived with the faulty belief that all the child-related recommendations offered by respected health organizations would be the most rigorously studied and *safest* available. If something terrible and tragic resulted from these recommendations, I thought, it would have to happen to one in a million children. This turned out not to be the case at all.

The hospital protocol for newborn breastfeeding management is called the Baby-Friendly Hospital Initiative (BFHI), a policy established in 1991 and guided by the WHO Ten Steps to Successful Breastfeeding guidelines.[2] This policy results in complications like dehydration, jaundice, or hypoglycemia, requiring extended or repeat hospitalization, for 5–16 percent of exclusively breastfed newborn babies worldwide.[3] And, as Dr. Vinod Bhutani, the leading newborn-jaundice expert, writes, "In the presence of early discharge (<48 hours age), successful promotion of breastfeeding and other risk factors . . . a small but apparently increasing number of babies experience severe hyperbilirubinemia [jaundice from high levels of bilirubin, a breakdown product of red blood cells that can accumulate in the blood due to insufficient feeding] that results in profound and permanent neurologic [brain] damage."[4]

Some infants experience complications that resolve undetected when a mother decides to give her hungry baby supplementation. Others are brought back to the hospital lethargic and unable to feed by bewildered parents who were simply following what their health professionals said was best for their child. Some of these newborns suffer complications severe enough to cause irreversible brain injury and long-term disability. My firstborn son was one of them.

Almost four years later, my son was diagnosed with intellectual disabilities, sensory processing disorder, autism, severe language impairment, fine and gross motor delays, coordination and gait abnormalities, and a seizure disorder. Since his diagnosis, I have researched the medical literature on starvation-related complications while breastfeeding and the brain injury and developmental disabilities that can result. The medical literature on these complications—newborn jaundice,[5] hypernatremic dehydration,[6] and hypoglycemia[7]—uniformly recognizes these complications as known causes of perinatal brain injury, intellectual impairment, attention deficit, motor/auditory/visual deficits, speech and language impairments, seizure disorders, and behavioral problems.[8] The AAP and the Academy of Breastfeeding Medicine (ABM) have guidelines to detect and treat these known complications, yet few parents are informed that they can occur during the course of exclusive breastfeeding.[9]

When I would eventually share my story with friends, family, and colleagues in my community and on social media, many shared stories of their own babies' complications while exclusively breastfeeding, some of whom showed developmental delays and disabilities years after. These stories often involved mothers who were conscientious and highly educated, read breastfeeding books, and were motivated to exclusively breastfeed. These mothers were taught to avoid formula, that insufficient breast milk was rare, and that frequent crying and nursing were normal and necessary to bring in their full milk supply. Most of all, their breastfeeding resources had instilled in them a fear of formula—that even one bottle would set their infant up for a lifetime of health problems like asthma, allergies, diabetes, lower IQ, leukemia, and even sudden infant death,[10] when a closer look at the scientific literature shows that there is no causal relationship between supplemental feedings and these conditions, and that the associations between long-term formula feeding and these health conditions are either conflicting, weak, or nonexistent when other factors are considered (as we'll see in chapter three).[11] These resources told parents that supplementation would cause their breastfeeding relationship to fail (and, by proxy, make them a failure as a mother), when clinical trials show no such relationship.[12] By hiding the possibility of insufficient breast milk intake and emphasizing the dangers of formula, trusted sources of breastfeeding education were leading parents to avoid supplementation even when their babies showed signs of needing it. As a result, children could go days—even weeks or months—underfed, until parents find them difficult to wake, dehydrated, malnourished, and in need of hospital admission.

When nurses and physicians I knew confirmed that these complications happened to babies routinely, I was shocked and horrified. It became obvious that trusted sources of health information were failing parents abysmally by not educating them on critical matters of infant feeding. Why was this happening, when teaching the importance of supplementing hungry babies could potentially save millions of children from these horrible and preventable outcomes?

In 2015, the first paper describing the devastating effects of hypoglycemia in poorly fed, previously healthy full-term breastfed newborns was published in *Hospital Pediatrics*.[13] The article described eleven exclusively breastfed newborn babies who developed profound hypoglycemia two to five days after birth from insufficient breast milk intake. One child was a healthy full-term baby who presented just like my son. Despite being seen by the pediatrician on the third day, he was found lethargic and unable to feed on the fourth day. He had lost 10 percent of his birth weight and had a low glucose of 20 mg/dL (normal > 47 mg/dL). The child was given IV glucose, after which he developed a seizure. A brain MRI showed extensive areas of injury affecting almost the entire brain. Ten other term-breastfed newborns were similarly found lethargic, seizing, hypothermic, and/or not breathing from hypoglycemia. Out of the six newborns who had received MRIs, five showed widespread brain injury in varying patterns. These children subsequently developed long-term disabilities, including seizure disorders, motor weakness, visual impairment, and feeding difficulties requiring speech therapy.

What I had suspected from my child's story and my research on breastfeeding complications was confirmed. How many babies have been injured in the same way—and why aren't parents being warned? While certainly not all cases of insufficient breast milk intake result in developmental disabilities, the fact that it is a known risk should make informing parents on how to prevent it a top priority.

As a physician and a mother discovering a serious and preventable patient safety hazard, I wrote to several medical authorities, expecting that they would be alarmed and promptly alert new parents. I wrote to the AAP, the CDC, the Joint Commission (a hospital safety organization), and even the authors of the breastfeeding book that I read. In their email response, it was apparent that the book authors were oblivious to the serious, well-documented, long-term consequences of what happened to my son. I received minimal response from the health organizations. No alarm was sounded.

THE BIRTH OF FED IS BEST

That's when I began publicly sharing my story on social media. It reached millions across the globe. Parents and health professionals also started posting their own stories. Since then, I have collected tens of thousands of breastfeeding stories from parents on social media. I discovered that parents and health professionals have been witnessing these complications for decades, and that health authorities have done little to alert the public. I learned that my son's story is not unique, and that a version of his story is happening every single day in hospitals around the globe that follow the WHO Baby-Friendly protocol. Yet few parents are told it could happen until they experience it themselves.

During the process of reaching millions, I was fortunate to find Jody Segrave-Daly, a neonatal intensive care unit (NICU) nurse and IBCLC. She is an expert in infant feeding, having worked in newborn nurseries and newborn intensive care units for the better part of three decades and later founded a private practice that assisted parents and babies with lactation and feeding challenges in the community.

Jody had been in the position of starting life-saving IV lines on the tiny collapsed veins of dehydrated newborns many times, and comforting traumatized mothers who had just discovered that they had inadvertently starved their child while following the exclusive breastfeeding guidelines. Since 2013, she had observed an alarming increase in the number of breastfed infants requiring admission for dehydration, hyperbilirubinemia, and hypoglycemia due to underfeeding, as well as babies requiring rescue supplementation during home consultations due to delayed onset of full milk production. And as a seasoned NICU nurse, as well as a mother who successfully breastfed her three children, she had significant concerns about the lactation education being taught to health professionals—especially how the risks of insufficient feeding were being omitted and how to prevent them with education and temporary supplementation.

Other lactation consultants (LCs) had contacted me as well with the same concerns but had asked to remain anonymous for fear of backlash from the LC community. They wanted to do something to improve protocols so that no baby would be put at risk due to failure to act on early signs of insufficient milk intake. They wanted to destigmatize the use of infant formula as a preventive tool when human milk was inadequate. Most of all, they wanted mothers to be *believed* when they expressed concern that their babies were hungry.

In response to this public health crisis, Jody and I cofounded the Fed Is Best Foundation, a 501(c)(3) nonprofit organization, on July 11, 2016. Today, the Foundation consists of a network of volunteer doctors, nurses, lactation consultants, parents, and patient advocates who study the science of infant-feeding complications and advocate for safe infant-feeding practices. The foundation's social media platform provides direct comprehensive support to all parents, whether breastfeeding, combination-feeding, formula-feeding, or tube-feeding. Our Facebook page has built a following of almost a million around the globe.

After my story went viral, we met Lynnette Hafken, MA, an IBCLC and former La Leche League Leader, whose longtime passion was helping parents nurse their babies—regardless of how much milk they produce. After being deeply moved by my son's story, she reached out with her own concerns about the rigidity in current breastfeeding advocacy that, for far too many families, has resulted in babies failing to thrive, parental trauma, and, ironically, premature cessation of breastfeeding. She is now director of support services for the Foundation, supporting mothers and colleagues through our online groups and contributing heavily to our educational and advocacy material.

Eventually the news media began to catch wind of our organization's work. On February 25, 2017, we published the story of Landon Johnson, who was born in a Southern California Baby-Friendly–certified hospital. Landon showed signs of distress, namely nonstop crying and nursing for more than forty-eight hours while in the hospital. His mother, Jillian Johnson, who was educated by the hospital's breastfeeding class and encouraged by her health professionals to exclusively breastfeed, was told repeatedly that this behavior was normal. He had produced the expected number of wet and dirty diapers and was discharged at around 9.7 percent weight loss with next day follow-up. There was no recommendation for supplemental feedings.

Twelve hours after discharge, Landon was found unresponsive, in cardiac arrest from severe dehydration. He was diagnosed with hypernatremic dehydration, a complication of insufficient feeding in exclusively breastfed newborns. He died nineteen days later, once it was determined he had suffered extensive brain injury from dehydration and cardiac arrest, and he was taken off life support.

This story was read over a million times in four days. Media organizations asked to interview us and Jillian Johnson regarding these events and Landon's story, and Fed Is Best received global media attention. We were also invited on *The Doctors*, where Jillian and I shared our stories and advocated for safe infant-feeding education.[14]

Since then, we have been interviewed by dozens of media outlets, including CNN,[15] *TIME* magazine,[16] the *Washington Post*,[17] *People* magazine, the *New York Times*, the CBC in Canada,[18] and the BBC,[19] to name a few. The *New York Times* invited Jody to write "How to Breastfeed During the First Two Weeks of Life"[20] and contribute to "How to Deal with Low Breastmilk Supply."[21] Celebrities, television shows, and hundreds of news articles have affirmed the "Fed Is Best" mantra, recognizing that not all parents can or choose to breastfeed and that making sure a baby and their parents are healthy and happy is the most important goal of infant feeding. Senior members of Fed Is Best have spoken at hospitals, national medical conferences, the National Institutes of Health, and the US Department of Agriculture.[22] Several pediatricians have since published their own criticisms of the BFHI policies in news outlets, medical journals, and conferences.[23]

MEETING WITH THE WORLD HEALTH ORGANIZATION

Around this time, Julie Tibbets joined us as our pro bono attorney and arranged a meeting with the top officials of the WHO's infant-feeding division, Dr. Nigel Rollins and Dr. Laurence Grummer-Strawn. On September 22, 2017, the physicians and nurses of the Fed Is Best Foundation, including Tibbets and guest expert Dr. Paul Thornton, the lead author of the Pediatric Endocrine Society's neonatal hypoglycemia guidelines, met with the WHO officials to discuss the issue of newborn-feeding complications resulting from the Baby-Friendly Hospital Initiative policies.[24] I asked the officials what they knew about the percentage of infants developing feeding complications under Baby-Friendly policies. Surprisingly, they stated that the question felt "unfair" and ultimately provided no answer. They said that they had not specifically studied the negative effects of the Initiative and had commissioned no grants to study or monitor complications of the BFHI—that they mostly relied on available published peer-reviewed studies. They said that they had convened a group of global infant nutrition experts in the past year to review and revise its guidelines, but no one had raised the issue of complications as a priority for discussion.

I provided a slide presentation describing the number of breastfed newborns who were developing dehydration, jaundice, excessive weight loss, and hypoglycemia, and how many were at risk for preventable developmental impairments. A neonatologist present at the meeting, who has asked to be anonymous, recounted what neonatologists were seeing with the BFHI: breastfed infants who developed varying combinations of these complications and related brain injury due to the pressure to meet goals driven by hospital metrics around avoiding formula supplementation. Drawing from discussion with dozens of neonatologists regarding their experiences with the BFHI, she stated, "Neonatologists are seeing these cases almost every day everywhere around the country. The focus is only on the number of women who are exclusively breastfeeding at discharge and not at all on safety. [Exclusive] breastfeeding is the core measure and that's it!"[25]

When I asked the officials point-blank, "Are there any plans within the WHO to inform mothers of the risks of brain injury from insufficient breast milk, in order to make sure that they are aware, when a child is critically ill at home, that supplementation can protect their child from brain injury?" Dr. Rollins responded, "That specific recommendation, that was not identified by the experts in the guideline's scoping as a top priority."

Why not? "Within the guidelines," he continued, "there is literature in general on the danger signs, things like convulsions, being lethargic and not being able to feed. Those are clinical signs that are routinely included in materials taught to healthcare workers and when health workers communicate to mothers. Those signs are identified as 'alert' signs.

"The difficult thing," Dr. Rollins continued, "is that there are many things that cause those signs—it's not a singular cause. Any child demonstrating those signs needs a true workup in order to try and figure out exactly what's there. The signs that need assessment to identify the underlying cause are firmly there within the WHO guidelines."[26]

There was shocked silence at this response. The WHO was aware of the danger signs that signaled insufficient feeding complications that can result in brain injury. They confirmed that health professionals trained in the Baby-Friendly policy are taught to look for these signs. They knew these complications could happen at home where no health monitoring was available. But they had no plans to *fully inform* parents of the consequences of brain injury from inadequate feeding and that it could be prevented with supplementation. Parents are currently told some signs of these complications on their discharge instructions, to meet the hospital's minimal medico-legal obligation, but are not given enough education to know they stem from insufficient breast milk, and that supplementation can protect their children.

I felt like I was witnessing a crime. As a physician who has taken an oath to protect the health and safety of every individual, I was witnessing my colleagues—top officials whose influence had global reach—say that they effectively withhold information about a serious and preventable safety risk from parents who trusted them for advice regarding their child's health.

Despite this disappointing meeting, increasing public recognition of the problems with the "Breast Is Best" campaign has resulted in some policy changes. In August 2017, the Australian Medical Association updated its position statement on infant feeding, stating that "Parents who are unable or choose not to breastfeed should be provided with appropriate care and assistance to formula feed their child."[27] In June 2018, the Royal College of Midwives in the United Kingdom published a new position statement confirming that "the decision of whether or not to breastfeed is a woman's choice and must be respected," adding that "We recognize that some women cannot or do not wish to breastfeed and rely on formula milk. They must be given all the advice and support they need on safe preparation of bottles and responsive feeding to develop a close and loving bond with their baby."[28] In October 2018, the American College of Obstetricians and Gynecologists also amended their position on breastfeeding, stating, "Obstetrician–gynecologists and other obstetric care providers should support each woman's informed decision about whether to initiate or continue breastfeeding, recognizing that she is uniquely qualified to decide whether exclusive breastfeeding, mixed feeding, or formula feeding is optimal for her and her infant."[29]

On January 1, 2019, the Joint Commission, a US hospital-safety oversight organization, published a new perinatal core measure called "PC-06: Unexpected Complications in Term Newborns" that requires hospitals to report their rates of unexpected negative outcomes in healthy term newborns. These include severe neurological complications, severe shock and resuscitation, and hyperbilirubinemia requiring phototherapy. They state that this core measure serves to balance out potential adverse outcomes of other core measures. Measuring hyperbilirubinemia and phototherapy rates are particularly important, as the fifth perinatal core measure is exclusive breastfeeding before hospital discharge, which increases the risk of hyperbilirubinemia.[30]

After years of negative press, on December 3, 2019, Baby-Friendly USA, the organization that certifies US Baby-Friendly hospitals, published a blog entitled "What SHOULD Happen When Baby Does Not Get Enough Milk from Mom." The question was answered by pediatricians Dr. Casey Rosen-Carole, MD, MPH, MEd, lead author of the ABM's supplementation guidelines, and Dr. Bobbi Philipp, MD.[31] Dr. Rosen-Carole wrote:

Delayed lactogenesis [full milk production] is actually increasingly common because the risk factors for it are potentially increasing. When a baby is born into that situation, the goal is to closely monitor what the baby is doing, instead of giving a bottle right away . . . [but] if the baby is hungry and they're not getting enough milk out of the mother's breast, then they need to be supplemented. If lactogenesis [milk coming in] hasn't happened and you're at day 2 or 3 and the baby is not acting full at the breast, they have excess weight loss, or they are not peeing or pooping appropriately, then I think every breastfeeding expert is going to agree that it's time to develop an infant feeding plan that includes supplementation.

Dr. Philipp agreed, stating, "If you see signs that the mother's milk is insufficient, you need to feed the baby."

There was further acknowledgment of the dangers of dismissing signs of insufficient feeding by Trish McEnroe, executive director of Baby-Friendly USA,[32] who was asked by the *New York Times* in January 2020 about infants harmed by Baby-Friendly policies. She stated that "these stories are heartbreaking. Safety is the first priority. If a step can't be done safely, it shouldn't be done." It is tragic that only years after Fed Is Best started publishing these stories were we finally hearing what should have been the standard all along.

On September 1, 2020, the US Healthy People 2030 Goals, which sets national benchmarks for health promotion, removed the goals of reducing formula supplementation in the first two days after birth and of increasing the number of Baby-Friendly–certified hospitals.[33] Finally, on August 2, 2021, the Centers for Medicare & Medicaid Services announced that they would remove the exclusive metric of breast milk feeding rate at discharge when determining hospital reimbursements, a financial incentive that has put pressure on hospitals to discourage formula supplementation even when signs of persistent infant hunger occur.

After a few years of advocacy and community outreach, Fed Is Best has changed the infant-feeding discourse and global health policies. In the process, it has amassed a large collection of stories, research, and resources to support all families and all forms of safe infant feeding. Our resources use the most up-to-date research to answer many questions that are glaringly absent from many infant-feeding resources: How much breast milk and/or formula a day is required to keep an infant safely fed? What bilirubin, sodium, and glucose levels—the biological markers of starvation and dehydration—increase the risk of developmental disabilities?

But while we have come a long way, we continue to receive stories of breastfed infants needing hospital admission because they didn't receive enough milk. Hospital guidelines continue to inadequately monitor and protect infants from complications while poorly protecting them from conditions associated with moderate cognitive impairment.[34] Parent educational resources often don't give parents clear criteria for when supplementation is necessary *before* medical complications arise.

THIS BOOK'S MISSION

Which leads us to the *Fed Is Best* book, a chronicle of infant-feeding history, policy, and beliefs, and an inclusive, evidence-based guide to safe infant feeding. This book represents several years and thousands of hours of research into the scientific literature on infant feeding, parents' stories, and the clinical experiences of health professionals who care for infants. We answer many questions and give families realistic expectations so that they can be prepared for when the unexpected occurs. Breastfeeding is one major topic in healthcare where families are *not* provided all the information they need to keep their children safe and healthy, and we intend to give you that information.

The fundamental truth of infant feeding is that children who are safely fed enough fluid, nutrients, and calories thrive, and those who are not fed enough or are fed unsafe substitutes have poorer health and brain development—and when there are no safe alternatives, they die. Part 1 of this book reviews the history and science of infant feeding, including information on an infant's nutritional requirements for optimal brain development.

Part 2 provides detailed information on how to tell if your baby is getting the nutrition they need. A significant portion of this book is dedicated to helping parents who wish to breastfeed succeed by providing realistic and sustainable solutions if problems arise. We teach how to fully recognize hunger and satisfaction cues, estimate milk supply, monitor weight, interpret blood work related to feeding, and determine whether supplementation is needed. We do this while teaching how to maintain and maximize milk supply and continued latching during supplementation. We teach breastfeeding differently by prioritizing the goal of safe and adequate feeding and by destigmatizing the use of supplemental formula (or banked donor breast milk if available) when a parent sees that their baby needs it—*before* it becomes a medical problem. We do so to help protect an infant's human right to be fully fed, so that they can reach their full potential.

Part 2 also gives necessary attention to less talked-about forms of infant feeding, like combination feeding and exclusive formula feeding, so that families who need or choose them can also ensure their babies are healthy and thriving. QR codes throughout lead to printable online resources like the Fed Is Best Feeding Plan, newborn weight loss and growth charts, daily milk calculators, and much more. And for the many special feeding circumstances that require equal attention, like tube feeding and other medical conditions, you can find more information online at fedisbestbook. org, also accessible via the QR code.

Through *Fed Is Best,* we hope to offer a perspective that makes ideal infant feeding available to *everyone*, regardless of a mother and baby's ability to breastfeed. By showing how common it is to struggle with infant feeding, we also hope to foster greater understanding and respect for the diversity of human circumstances that determine what "best" infant feeding looks like. We thus hope to counter the parent shaming that has become too common in modern parenting discourse. Our mantra is a long-awaited message that families and health professionals alike have embraced. Ultimately, we hope to restore humanity, reason, and choice to the world of infant feeding and remind everyone that the first rule of nature is and has *always* been that "Fed Is Best."

—Christie del Castillo-Hegyi, MD

THE TAKE-HOME POINTS

For Tired Parents Needing
the Bottom Line

For any new parents struggling to feed their babies—who also may be sleep deprived from the challenges of early parenthood—if there is one thing you need to learn from this book, it is this:

> **The most important rule of infant feeding is *feed your baby*,
> whether with human milk, infant formula, or both.**

Infant health and brain development are optimal when they are fed *all* the calories, fluid, and nutrients they need from birth into adulthood. We are all bound by the laws of biology, which require us to continuously provide our living cells with oxygen, fluid, and nutrients to maintain their survival and proper functioning. No study has ever shown that depriving infants of their daily nutritional requirements—as happens when insufficient colostrum or mature breast milk is produced—is beneficial to infant health. In fact, quite the opposite is true.

If you can and want to breastfeed your baby, your efforts should be supported *in every way possible*, while you ensure your baby receives all the nutrition they need to ensure optimal health and development. If you

17

wish to feed a combination of breast milk and formula, want to exclusively
formula-feed, or need to tube-feed your child (if medical conditions prevent
oral feeding), you should be supported in achieving these goals. Period.
How can we ensure optimal nutrition for all babies? *By listening to them.*
**By listening to our own parental instincts and supplementing when
necessary—an instinct that has protected infants from malnutrition
for millennia.** As long as your baby is being safely and sufficiently fed with
love, you have not failed.

How do you know when your baby is still hungry and whether they
need additional nutrition to keep them safely fed? If your newborn is crying
nonstop, latching then crying even after nursing, and breastfeeding for longer than thirty to forty-five minutes, every one to two hours, for more than
four hours, or even continuously—especially if your milk is not yet in—
your baby is hungry and needs more breast milk or formula. If your baby is
sleepy all the time or difficult to wake, or has trouble keeping awake during
feedings, your baby may not be getting enough calories to feed well. In both
cases, supplement your baby until they're full, with banked donor milk or
formula, whichever is available, and see your baby's doctor right away.

Nothing is more important to your baby's health and future than getting fed. You are not a failure if you need to supplement with formula.
More often than not, your baby will still go on to breastfeed successfully,
like millions of newborns have before. Parents have been supplementing
breastfeeding for millennia to buffer the effects of imperfect breast milk
supply. You are also not a failure if you cannot produce milk at all or if you
choose to formula-feed. You are providing your child what they need to *not
go hungry,* an act that, on its own, contributes far more to their health and
future than perhaps anything else you can do as a parent.

There are many "best" forms of infant feeding, and they include
exclusive breastfeeding, combination feeding, exclusive formula feeding,
exclusive pumped-milk feeding, and tube feeding. Given wide variations
in breast milk supply; breast and infant anatomy; infant latching ability;
and physical, psychological, occupational, and social conditions, the form
of feeding that is best for a baby will be different for every family. From

the authors of this book—a physician, a nurse/LC, and an LC—who have received thousands of stories of tragedies resulting from the cruel falsehood that needing formula is "failure" or even harmful, you are hereby given permission to *use your own judgment to determine whether your infant-feeding plan is working* . . . because at the end of the day, *you* are the person best positioned to know what is best. No other "best" matters.

PART 1
The History and Science of Infant Feeding

1

Breastfeeding and Bottle Feeding from 1550 BC to Today

The true history of breastfeeding and bottle feeding can be boiled down to the following: there have always been mothers who produced plenty of breast milk, and there have always been mothers who did not. As a matter of natural selection, children of mothers with abundant milk supply thrived, enjoyed better health and brain development, and suffered from fewer infectious diseases related to contaminated sources of nutrition. Children of mothers who lacked sufficient supply commonly did not, unless they had access to safe alternatives.[1] Infants communicate that a mother's breast milk is not enough by crying until they are fed; parents across the globe have responded to these cries by finding alternatives to prevent hunger and starvation. Parents have supplemented breastfeeding when breast milk supply is insufficient for millennia, and it is part of our human evolution: it allowed infants who would have starved from insufficient breast milk to survive and thrive into adulthood.

Knowing the history of breastfeeding, lactation failure, wet nursing, and bottle feeding is vital for understanding how past humans responded to the problem of insufficient breast milk. This struggle is not new; although the pendulum of public opinion has swung wildly over time, *fed* has always been best.

LACTATION INSUFFICIENCY, EARLY BREAST MILK SUBSTITUTES, AND THE RISE OF FORMULA FEEDING

According to "The History of Infant Feeding," published in the *Journal of Perinatal Education,* one of the earliest written records of lactation failure occurred in 1550 BC, as published in "The Papyrus Ebers" from Egypt:[2] "To get a supply of milk in a woman's breast for suckling a child: warm the bones of a sword fish in oil and rub her back with it." But the authors noted that, as early as 2000 BC in Israel, although breastfeeding was considered a religious obligation, it was recognized that it was not always possible, such as when the mother died during childbirth or lactation was inadequate.[3] Wet nursing, where other lactating women fed infants when their own mothers did not have enough, was the primary alternative. This practice began as early as 2000 BC and extended into the twentieth century.[4]

If wet nursing was not available, parents fed babies milk from domesticated animals. Infant-feeding vessels—small clay pots with spouts containing chemical evidence of milk from ruminant animals (like cows)—dating back to 5500–4800 BC have been found, according to recent research published in the journal *Nature.*[5] According to the author, "The fact that we can feed human babies animal milk for the first time means essentially that prehistoric women can have more babies, which sets us on the pathway to how we live today."[6] Animal milk substitutes came from goats, sheep, donkeys, camels, pigs, and horses, but mostly cows.

Unfortunately, before the wide availability of pasteurization, sanitation, and refrigeration, this practice was far more perilous to infants, given the high risk of contamination of animal milk and feeding vessels. Up to the eighteenth century, feeding bottles and makeshift teats were difficult to clean. According to a 1993 historical review, "In the early 19th century, the use of dirty feeding devices, combined with the lack of proper milk storage and sterilization, led to the death of *one-third* of all artificially fed infants during their first year of life" (italics added).[7] This gives us insight into the issue facing mothers and infants throughout human history: lactation insufficiency has always been a problem, and the alternatives to direct breastfeeding were limited or hazardous.

As sanitation and sterilization improved, the risks of bottle feeding decreased. Glass bottles and rubber nipples were developed during the mid-nineteenth century. With improved bottle cleaning and sterilization procedures and the advent of milk pasteurization, bottle feeding became a viable alternative to breastfeeding. In 1835, William Newton patented sterilized canned milk, also known as "evaporated milk," which provided a safer option for supplementation. But this alternative was limited in its nutritional value, as animal milk lacks many essential nutrients present in breast milk.

So, scientists began to develop vitamin-fortified cow's milk, now known as infant formula. In 1865, chemist Justus von Liebig developed and patented the first formula, which came in liquid form.[8] Multiple brands of formula became available, but they lacked essential vitamins, minerals, and protein required for optimal nutrition. However, given the reality of lactation insufficiency for many mothers, there was continued demand for better breast milk alternatives, which in turn led to advances in breast milk research and the development of formula that more closely mimics breast milk.

As expected of any successful product, the business of formula grew along with its marketing.[9] By 1929, the American Medical Association formed the Committee on Foods to ensure safety and quality of formula products.[10] For the first time, there was a safe alternative to breastfeeding, and formula companies created advertisements intended to promote formula feeding as the *best* solution. Formula was advertised directly to consumers and physicians as a modern, scientific, and superior choice to breastfeeding. Formula companies, most infamously the Nestlé Corporation, promoted formula as "Best for Babies," offering free samples upon request. Formula advertisements changed public attitudes, and soon formula feeding

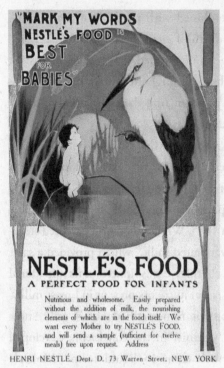

NESTLÉ'S FOOD

A PERFECT FOOD FOR INFANTS

Nutritious and wholesome. Easily prepared without the addition of milk, the nourishing elements of which are in the food itself. We want every Mother to try NESTLÉ'S FOOD, and will send a sample (sufficient for twelve meals) free upon request. Address

HENRI NESTLÉ. Dept. D. 73 Warren Street. NEW YORK

Nestlé directly advertised its product to consumers as a "perfect food for infants," offering free samples upon request.

became the primary mode of infant feeding in industrialized countries.[11] By the 1940s and 1950s, formula-feeding rates were increasing and breastfeeding rates were steadily decreasing, a trend that continued until the 1970s. The breastfeeding rate dropped from 90 percent in the nineteenth century to 42 percent in the twentieth century.[12]

As the formula industry grew in high-income countries, formula marketing extended into low- and middle-income countries (LMICs).[13] In addition to its misleading ads promoting formula as superior to breastfeeding, Nestlé more egregiously deployed sales representatives dressed as nurses to promote formula to communities, thus misrepresenting the product as something health professionals advocated. Nestlé also developed close relationships with clinics and hospitals and gave mothers free samples upon discharge from hospitals postbirth.[14] Most mothers were not counseled on the effects of replacing breastfeeding with formula on milk supply, and without appropriate breastfeeding management, formula feeding often led to less time breastfeeding and less milk removal. This resulted in reduced milk production, also known as secondary lactation failure,* and permanent reliance on formula.

---

* "Secondary failed lactation" means that the mother has the biological capacity to produce enough milk, yet mismanagement of breastfeeding has resulted in poor or absent milk production. This differs from "primary failed lactation," which has biological causes (such as insufficient glandular tissue).

Aggressive marketing of formula in the developing world led to global declines in breastfeeding rates, with devastating consequences to millions of infants in places where breastfeeding was the only safe and sustainable form of infant feeding.[15] Parents who lived in places with poor sanitation, whose children's survival relied heavily on a robust breast milk supply, would thus unwittingly expose their infants not only to the perils of insufficient breast milk but also to infections, as formula was often prepared with contaminated water and fed in unclean bottles.[16] Families often would not have the means to buy enough formula, so they diluted it to make it last longer. This led to infants dying or becoming critically ill from dehydration, malnutrition, and infectious diseases.[17] The National Bureau of Economic Research has estimated that millions of infants became ill and died because of this phenomenon.[18] The monetization of infant feeding by private corporations caused a tragic public health crisis.

THE RESURGENCE OF BREASTFEEDING AND THE WAR ON FORMULA

While breastfeeding declined in the United States, a small group of American women had become interested in sustaining the practice in their community. In 1956, La Leche League was formed in Franklin Park, Illinois, by a group of seven mothers who wanted to provide breastfeeding support to interested women.[19] Mary White and Marian Tompson enlisted the help of five of their friends and acquaintances, and the seven began holding monthly gatherings to discuss issues regarding pregnancy, childbirth, and breastfeeding. The organization grew and, in 1964, became La Leche League International, a global organization established to protect, support, and promote breastfeeding. In the 1970s, several more US breastfeeding advocacy groups formed, including the National Council of Churches' Interfaith Center on Corporate Responsibility and the Infant Formula Action Coalition, which began a public awareness campaign on the importance of breastfeeding. As a result, breastfeeding rates have steadily increased in the United States and the rest of the world.[20]

Pushback against the aggressive nature of formula marketing took hold in 1974, when a booklet called *The Baby Killer* was published by London's War on Want organization, exposing the Nestlé Corporation's predatory marketing practices in developing countries.[21] Through this campaign, the public became more aware of how the marketing of formula in the developing world was causing infant deaths from gastrointestinal illness and malnutrition. Global awareness of the Nestlé scandal ultimately led to the Nestlé boycott launched in 1977. This boycott not only galvanized the breastfeeding movement but once again changed public attitudes about breastfeeding and formula companies. Due to these companies' unethical actions, the tides began to turn against formula. And as we will see, the response to this public health emergency had unintended—and in some cases devastating—consequences.

In 1981, La Leche League International was given consultative status with UNICEF and subsequently was a major influence in the formation of the WHO/UNICEF breastfeeding policy.[22] In 1981, the International Code of Marketing of Breast-Milk Substitutes (the WHO Code) was adopted by the World Health Assembly of the World Health Organization, which codified restrictions on the marketing of breast milk substitutes, including infant formula, infant bottles, and nipples, to ensure that mothers were not discouraged from breastfeeding through predatory marketing practices. The code stipulated that there should be absolutely no promotion of breast milk substitutes and bottles, artificial nipples, or pacifiers to the public by health facilities or health professionals, and that free samples should not be provided to pregnant women, new mothers, or families.[23]

In 1989, under the consultation of La Leche League International, the WHO and UNICEF adopted the Ten Steps to Successful Breastfeeding,[24] which states that each healthcare facility providing maternity and newborn services should:

1.   have a written breastfeeding policy that is routinely communicated to all healthcare staff.
2.   train all healthcare staff in skills necessary to implement this policy.

3. inform all pregnant women about the benefits and management of breastfeeding.

4. help mothers initiate breastfeeding within half an hour of birth.

5. show mothers how to breastfeed, and how to maintain lactation even if they should be separated from their infants.

6. give newborn infants no food or drink other than breast milk, unless medically indicated.

7. practice rooming-in—that is, allow mothers and infants to remain together—twenty-four hours a day.

8. encourage breastfeeding on demand.

9. give no artificial nipples or pacifiers to breastfeeding infants.

10. foster the establishment of breastfeeding support groups and refer mothers to them on discharge from the hospital or clinic.

In 1990, WHO and UNICEF member states adopted the Innocenti Declaration to protect, promote, and support breastfeeding with the goal of promoting infant health and optimal nutrition.[25] Here are key quotes from the Declaration:

> All women should be enabled to practice exclusive breastfeeding and all infants should be fed exclusively on breast milk from birth to 4–6 months of age. Thereafter, children should continue to be breastfed, while receiving appropriate and adequate complementary foods, for up to two years of age or beyond.

> Attainment of [the Declaration's breastfeeding goals] requires . . . the reinforcement of a "breastfeeding culture" and its vigorous defense against incursions of a "bottle feeding culture" . . . utilizing to the full the prestige and authority of acknowledged leaders of society in all walks of life.

> Efforts should be made to increase women's confidence in their ability to breastfeed. Such empowerment involves the removal of

constraints and influences that manipulate perceptions and behavior towards breastfeeding, often by subtle and indirect means . . . [a] comprehensive communications strategy [is needed] involving all media and addressed to all levels of society.

• • •

All governments should develop national breastfeeding policies and set appropriate national targets for the 1990s. They should establish a national system for monitoring the attainment of their targets, and they should develop indicators such as the prevalence of exclusively breastfed infants at discharge from maternity services, and the prevalence of exclusively breastfed infants at four months of age.

• • •

Ensure that every facility providing maternity services fully practices all ten of the Ten Steps to Successful Breastfeeding set out in the joint WHO/UNICEF statement "Protecting, promoting and supporting breastfeeding . . ."

• • •

Take action to give effect to the principles and aim of all Articles of the International Code of Marketing of Breast-Milk Substitutes and subsequent relevant World Health Assembly resolutions in their entirety; and enacted legislation protecting the breastfeeding rights of working women and established means for its enforcement.

The wording of the Innocenti Declaration makes clear that this was a declaration intended not only to promote and increase global breastfeeding rates but also to promote breastfeeding *only*—thus discouraging mixed or exclusive formula feeding. It makes no mention about the reality of what happens when breastfeeding is not enough, which women have always faced. Women's opinions and choices are assumed to stem from lack of confidence or education, or manipulated perceptions, rather than valid observations of inadequate milk supply. The Declaration also specifically calls out tenets of what would become the Ten Steps to Successful Breastfeeding as the method through which breastfeeding would be promoted.

In 1991, the Baby-Friendly Hospital Initiative (BFHI), based on the Ten Steps to Successful Breastfeeding, was launched globally. This hospital accreditation program trains health facilities and families to follow the Ten Steps. The most important and effective part of the program is that it teaches the necessary skills for breastfeeding. However, it goes one step further by saying that almost all mothers should strive to breastfeed exclusively. This recommendation requires everyone to accept a very big and unsubstantiated assumption: that with proper management and unlimited nursing, all birthing mothers, with rare exceptions, will be able to produce enough milk to meet their infant's full nutritional requirement from birth to six months. It also ignores the possibility of significant problems stemming from recommending one single best way to feed infants in a world where mothers vary widely in their ability to produce milk.

As the BFHI spread to more hospitals, health professionals became aware of the complications plaguing exclusively breastfed infants whose parents were unwittingly underfeeding them while following the recommendations. Since then, pediatric health providers have widely recognized that insufficient feeding complications occur in a predictable number of exclusively breastfed infants, especially in the days before milk comes in. This is why the Academy of Breastfeeding Medicine developed guidelines to identify these infants with the hope of correcting feeding complications before brain injury occurs.[26] These guidelines recommended weight and bilirubin monitoring, with glucose monitoring on higher-risk infants, while parents were left largely unaware of the reason why they were done: to identify underfed babies.

The new standard of promoting exclusive breastfeeding for almost all newborns made it necessary to set standards for safe and acceptable weight loss and bilirubin and glucose levels to determine when it would be "medically indicated" to supplement with formula. The goal was to avoid formula and maintain exclusive breastfeeding status for as many infants as possible, while preventing conditions that could impair brain development.

Unfortunately, such a system necessarily missed some who would be supplemented too late, especially when these complications occur at home, since parents were left unaware of the possibility or signs of underfeeding. Additionally, these supplementation guidelines were largely based on the "expert opinion" of the guidelines' makers, not on prospective studies proving their safety.

Since the launch of the BFHI, world breastfeeding rates have in fact increased dramatically, particularly in high-income countries. What has also increased worldwide are hospital admissions for insufficient-feeding complications—namely, jaundice and dehydration—in breastfed newborns. Today, these are the leading causes of full-term newborn readmissions across the globe.[27] To dissect how we got here, we must discuss the current breastfeeding paradigm, what tenets have been disproven by science, and what widely circulating myths are harming a significant portion of infants and families.

2

Another Look at What We Are Taught About Breastfeeding

According to the WHO, "As a global public health recommendation, infants should be exclusively breastfed for the first six months of life to achieve optimal growth, development and health," and "exclusive breastfeeding from birth is possible except for a few medical conditions, and unrestricted exclusive breastfeeding results in ample milk production."[1] We are taught that it is "rare" to have a true biological limitation to milk production, and hence supplementation is rarely needed. Maternal reports of low milk supply due to frequent or constant crying and nursing (which are in fact common signs of persistent hunger) are often cast as inaccurate interpretations of "normal" infant behavior, called *"perception of insufficient milk"* (PIM) or *"self-reported insufficient milk"* (SRIM) in scientific journals. Low milk supply is primarily blamed on misperception and miseducation of parents, manipulated perceptions due to formula ads or a "bottle-feeding culture," inadequate lactation support, poor maternal

33

effort, mismanagement by health professionals, birth interventions, and inappropriate formula supplementation. Rarely is biology cited as a cause.

Breastfeeding resources recommend that formula be avoided from the moment of birth unless there is a medical indication. The first milk a birthing parent produces is colostrum, which is present in small volumes per feed: about 5–7 mL on day 1, 10–20 mL on day 2, and 20–30 mL on day 3. Around day 4, when the full milk supply "comes in" (also known as lactogenesis II), the birthing parent begins producing mature milk, ideally in volumes greater than 60 mL per feed.[2] This transition is required to meet the full nutritional requirement of an exclusively breastfed baby. Parents and health professionals are taught that colostrum is more nutritionally dense than mature breast milk, and that despite its small volume, it provides *all* the nutrition a newborn needs. They say this is because a newborn's stomach is so tiny, about 5–7 mL on the first day, then growing by the same volume as colostrum transitions to mature milk, likewise reaching 60 mL (a tenfold growth of an organ in a matter of days). We are taught that feeding more than these volumes with formula will abnormally "stretch" the infant stomach and permanently predispose them to future obesity.

A central tenet of the exclusive-breastfeeding recommendation is that any introduction of formula will also reduce an infant's demand for direct breastfeeding. Advocates claim that if an infant is supplemented, they will invariably breastfeed less. Since human milk production works on a supply-and-demand basis, breastfeeding less would reduce the stimulus to make more milk, thus causing a downward spiral of milk production until the breasts stop making milk altogether (though as we will see, this is a misleading oversimplification).

A fully fed and hydrated newborn typically produces six to eight wet diapers and three or more dirty diapers a day, but it is normal before lactogenesis II for them to produce only one wet and one dirty diaper on day 1, two each on day 2, and three each on day 3.[3] Only when the milk comes in does the baby produce the full diaper count. After milk comes in, parents are taught, a baby can be sustained on breast milk alone until six months for all but a rare mother. As they grow, infants will increase their demand, signaling the breasts to produce more as needed. As long as a mother allows her infant to breastfeed as frequently and as long as they wish, parents are told, she *will* produce exactly what her baby needs.

This commonly depicted course of breastfeeding is often framed as the "biological norm." But what if the milk does not come in by day 3 and the baby continues to lose weight? Will they continue to get all they need from colostrum? How did researchers discover that nearly all women on the planet could produce exactly what their infants need through six months of age? How does a stomach grow tenfold over the course of three to four days? Why do so many exclusively breastfed (EBF) newborn babies cry so much until milk comes in? Why do they produce so few diapers, and why are they losing weight if they are really getting all that they need? If not producing enough milk is so rare, then why do so many mothers report problems with milk supply and say it is the reason they either supplement or stop breastfeeding altogether?

This widely disseminated story is in fact propped up with countless myths that do not match the reality of most birthing parents and infants. In fact, many of these claims are not supported by scientific data. The problem is, when myths about human biology and infant feeding are passed off as facts to parents and health professionals, they can have serious negative consequences to infant health and safety.

The following is not an exhaustive list of these myths and the inconvenient truths they obscure, but does include the major ones. As we'll see, when examined through scientific methods, these beliefs fall apart under the weight of objective evidence.

MYTH 1:

"It is rare to not produce enough milk to exclusively breastfeed."

Breastfeeding educational resources commonly claim that "only" 5 percent of mothers have true low breast milk supply.[4] To begin with, 5 percent (1 in 20) is *not* rare by any definition. So what is the actual number of mothers who have true low milk supply? Across thirty years of global exclusive-breastfeeding promotion, how many studies have measured the daily milk production of birthing mothers from birth to six months to know that nearly all will produce exactly what their infants need if they breastfeed on demand? Surely, such an important, universally applied recommendation would require several studies of at least tens of thousands of mothers to make sure all infants whose parents followed them would be adequately fed and healthy. **Yet there is not a single study measuring daily milk production from birth to six months to support this claim. Not one.**

All of the available data was collected by a WHO expert panel in a 2002 published review called "Nutrient Adequacy of Exclusive Breastfeeding for the Term Infant During the First Six Months of Life." This review was designed to assess whether nutrient intakes provided by human milk are sufficient to meet infant nutritional requirements defined by "growth, [and] other functional outcomes, e.g. immune response and neurodevelopment."[5] But the authors acknowledged that there were major limitations in making a universal six-month exclusive breastfeeding recommendation, as "exclusive breastfeeding at 6 months is not a common practice in developed countries, and it is *rarer still in developing countries*" (our emphasis) and that "the inability to estimate the proportion of exclusively breastfed infants at risk of specific deficiencies is a major drawback in terms of developing appropriate public health policies." They noted that there were "marked attrition rates in exclusive breastfeeding through 6 months postpartum, even among women who are both well-nourished and highly motivated."

In other words, even by their own account, the WHO's exclusive breastfeeding recommendation was *rarely practiced* anywhere and that even among healthy, motivated mothers, a significant portion did not or could not meet the six-month exclusive-breastfeeding goal. This rapid drop in exclusive-breastfeeding rates made it difficult to know when additional nutrition would be needed to meet an infant's need.

So, not only did the WHO panel lack data on the percentage of women who were physically unable to produce the amount of milk required to safely meet their baby's needs; it also lacked data on how many infants would become malnourished because of it. According to the panel, milk intake estimates were derived from "self-selected" populations; no "randomly representative data" was available. What this means is that the data was a snapshot of the milk production of mothers who were *already* successfully exclusively breastfeeding, not a random sample of the population to know how many *couldn't* exclusively breastfeed. Such data provides no information on whether—as the WHO claims—*most* mothers "with few exceptions" can safely achieve the exclusive-breastfeeding standard.

How many women have insufficient breast milk that makes exclusively breastfeeding unsafe or impossible? The largest study measuring the daily milk production of healthy mothers who were motivated to exclusively breastfeed and had close lactation management followed them only up to *one month*. It found that **two-thirds** of these mothers had less than the minimum 440 mL/day required to breastfeed exclusively by days 11 to 13, and **one-third** did at day 28.[6] While this study might have attracted more low-supply mothers to participate (as mothers with low supply are more motivated to put in the amount of effort required), thereby inflating the number with low supply, it's worth noting that the 440 mL daily minimum used by the study authors only meets the requirements of an average 6.5-pound (3 kg) newborn, and is not enough to support growth past this weight. This would *underestimate* the percent of low-supply mothers, as many infants weigh more than 3 kg. Therefore, according to the best study on breast milk production to date, problems with insufficient breast milk supply are quite common, even with good lactation management.

Another study, done by Dr. Marianne Neifert, lactation researcher and cofounder of the Academy of Breastfeeding Medicine (the organization that provides hospital breastfeeding guidelines for the BFHI), and colleagues found that among healthy, first-time mothers motivated to exclusively breastfeed who delivered term babies, 15 percent—or *more than 1 in 7*—at three weeks after delivery had persistent milk insufficiency despite "intensive intervention" by lactation professionals.[7]

Persistent milk insufficiency isn't the only issue breastfeeding parents face. Delayed onset of full milk production, also known as *delayed lactogenesis II* (DLII), is common, occurring in 22 percent of healthy mothers delivering full-term babies who were motivated to exclusively breastfeed and had LC support.[8] Two other studies show even higher rates of DLII (42% and 44%) among first-time mothers.[9] (Chapter five has a full list of DLII risk factors.) This data has been highlighted by Alison Stuebe, MD, former ABM president, who wrote an article stating that as many as **one in seven** breastfed newborns do in fact require supplementation and that previous beliefs that early supplementation is rarely needed were inaccurate.[10]

In the months after giving birth, 40–50 percent of US women and 60–90 percent of women internationally who wean prior to six months report "not producing enough milk" or "baby not satisfied with breast milk" as the primary reason.[11] Yet maternal reports of insufficient breast milk are commonly dismissed in parent and academic literature as unreliable "perceptions," given the widely accepted (and unsubstantiated) belief that insufficient breast milk is rare. WHO advisor Rafael Perez-Escamilla, PhD, has even written, "Some have hypothesized that self-reported insufficient milk is simply a socially accepted excuse that women give for explaining why they are not practicing what they know is recommended infant-feeding behavior."[12] But according to lactation researchers Neifert and colleagues, "Numerous reports of critical malnutrition, hypernatremic dehydration and severe failure to thrive among breastfed infants offset claims by some that insufficient milk is more often 'perceived' than real."[13]

All in all, the published data on these phenomena challenges one of the central tenets of the BFHI: that the vast majority of mothers can exclusively breastfeed from birth to six months with a few medical exceptions. Despite their best efforts to exclusively breastfeed, mothers who have DLII or persistent low milk supply are unable to do so without endangering their child. Mothers with low milk supply are often framed as poorly educated, easily duped by formula ads, mistaken in their perceptions of infant hunger, or—worse yet—lacking in the diligence required to achieve the "best" for their child.[14] And because of these myths, these mothers are left feeling like they are rare biological anomalies and failures as parents.

Mothers commonly report to us that they expressed concern about their infants not getting enough breast milk only to be reassured by their health providers that their infants' behavior was normal and that they should continue exclusively breastfeeding. Only when a child is medically ill or growing poorly, despite days to weeks of frequent and prolonged nursing, is a mother sometimes told her milk was not enough. Not believing maternal reports of insufficient milk while failing to measure objective data is a form of medical gaslighting that harms not only babies but parents as well. Such blanket reassurances have contributed to the countless stories we have received of infants requiring hospitalization for not getting enough breast milk and of parents being traumatized when they realize these reassurances and the actions they inspired were the cause. Health professionals' failure to recognize abnormal feeding behavior have even led to high-cost litigation related to brain injury from hypoglycemia and jaundice.[15]

Mothers with insufficient supply should not feel like they are failing if they have to partially or fully bottle-feed. True breast milk supply problems are in fact common, despite everything you might be told to the contrary.[16] Research shows these problems have biological underpinnings with multiple medical factors that are often out of anyone's control.[17] And by supplementing with formula to ensure their infants are well nourished, such parents are, by definition, giving their child the best chance of having optimal health and brain development.[18] An infant who is fully nourished with either breast milk, formula, or both will do better than any infant who becomes malnourished in a failed attempt to breastfeed exclusively. Despite this, the stigma against formula feeding has grown, and it is driving a rise in maternal postpartum depression and anxiety among mothers who cannot breastfeed (which we discuss in chapter three).[19]

MYTH 2:

"The newborn stomach is only 5–7 mL on the first day. Giving greater volumes stretches out the stomach and predisposes babies to obesity."

If you search "newborn stomach" on the internet, you will find a ubiquitous infographic depicting the "size of the newborn stomach" at day 1, day 3, day 7, and one month, corresponding to 5–7 mL, 22–27 mL, 45–60 mL, and 80–150 mL.[20] This suggests a four- to tenfold growth of a human organ within days—a scientific impossibility given that, at a typical rate of cell division, such organ growth takes weeks to months to accomplish.[21]

In fact, scientific research using ultrasound and direct measurement shows that the actual size of the full-term newborn stomach is around 20–30 mL.[22] The stomach is a J-shaped pouch within a tube that empties into the lower digestive tract during feeding in response to hormonal signals of hunger in babies, just as it does in adults.[23] Stomach emptying slows when the body sends signals of satisfaction. Therefore, many two- to three-day-old newborns can easily take a full 60 mL (2 fluid oz) feed once a mother's full milk supply comes in,[24] despite still having a 20–30 mL stomach.

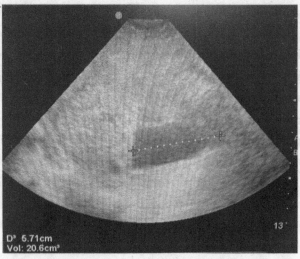

D³ 5.71cm
Vol: 20.6cm³

13

*Direct ultrasound measurement of term infant stomach in utero at 38 weeks, 4 days, measuring 20.6 mL.**

* It's important to note that while ultrasound estimates of fetal weight (which are derived from measurements of the infant head and femur) are often inaccurate, ultrasound can measure volume directly, whether in utero or after birth. Therefore, ultrasound measurements of the stomach volume are very accurate.

Summary of evidence on stomach capacity for human neonates

Author	Number	Method	Capacity
Goldstein et al. (1987)	152	Ultrasound	12 mL
Sase et al. (2000)	80	Ultrasound	-
Widstrom et al. (1988)*	25	Aspirates	10 mL
Zangen et al. (2001)	17	Balloon	20 mL
Scammon & Doyle (1920)	38	Autopsy	30–35 mL
Naveed et al. (1992)	100	Autopsy	18–20 mL
Kernesiuk et al. (1997)	11	Autopsy	15 mL
Bergman			20 mL

*This study, which instilled fluid into the stomach then aspirated (or sucked) it back out, likely underestimated the true volume of the newborn stomach, as some fluid would presumably advance into the lower gastrointestinal tract.

Table from a review combining the results of multiple studies measuring the newborn stomach size. No study shows a stomach size of 5–7 mL.

Does feeding more than the average colostrum volumes stretch out the stomach and cause obesity? When full milk supply comes in before forty-eight hours, mothers aren't told to limit feedings so they don't accidentally stretch out the newborn stomach; they are told to allow their baby to feed until they are satisfied. So why would formula distend the newborn stomach when breast milk supposedly doesn't? Because it is a fallacy. While there is some evidence that colostrum and breast milk may empty from the stomach a few minutes faster than formula, ultimately there is no evidence that "overfeeding" with either substance (feeding quantities greater than 30 mL) in the first days permanently "stretches out" the newborn stomach. The stomach is elastic, resuming its empty size as it empties into the lower intestinal tract, and it grows over weeks to months as the baby grows.

This brings us to the second part of this myth: that overfeeding with formula supplementation in the first days leads to obesity. What does science say? A 2020 study on the effects of "overfeeding" on the first day of life in formula-fed newborns looked at whether it increased rates of childhood overweight or obesity. They reviewed medical charts to see how many times babies were "overfed" (defined as being fed more than 30 mL of formula) and looked at well-child weight checks in the five years following. The article summary shared alarming information that these overfeeds had significantly increased rates of overweight and obesity. Yet the data showed only children in three categories—infants who received five, six, and seven overfeeds on the first day of life—had a statistically significant increased rate of being overweight at four years of age. And by the time they reached age five, all those differences in rates of being overweight disappeared! This makes this finding clinically meaningless.

Likewise, a 2018 study that looked at brief formula supplementation in breastfed neonates and the risk of being overweight at one year found supplementation did not affect rates of being overweight.[25] In fact, the largest study (called the PROBIT, which we detail in chapter three) on the effects of the BFHI-based EBF promotion, the cornerstone of which is avoidance of supplementation unless medically necessary, found that not only did BFHI-based intervention fail to lower rates of adolescent overweight and obesity, but that overweight and obesity rates were in fact statistically higher among those who received BFHI intervention.[26]

This is embarrassingly poor data, and yet breastfeeding parents continue to be told to avoid or limit supplementation for their persistently hungry newborns with the fallacy that it may cause obesity as justification. Regardless of the size of the newborn stomach, at the end of the day, the only one who truly knows what a baby needs to be satisfied is the baby.

MYTHS 3, 4, AND 5:

"Colostrum is more nutritionally dense than mature milk and it is all that a newborn needs for the first days." "Frequent crying and nursing are normal newborn behavior until milk comes in." "Newborn weight loss is caused by fluid shifts, not inadequate feeding."

Parents are commonly taught that colostrum is more nutritionally dense than mature milk and therefore can meet a newborn's full caloric requirement for several days until milk comes in.[27] Human milk research measuring the total caloric content of colostrum shows that, in fact, **colostrum has fewer calories than mature milk**, containing 54 calories* (kcal) per deciliter (dL) versus mature milk's 66 kcal/dL, or 16 versus 20 calories per oz, respectively.[28] While colostrum contains immunological components, according to human milk researchers, "the concentration of lactose . . . is low in colostrum, thus explaining the low volume of colostrum that is secreted and also indicating that the primary function of colostrum is to be immunological rather than nutritional."[29]

So, how much of the caloric requirement of a newborn is met by exclusive colostrum feeding?

We are about to tell you something you will rarely find in a breastfeeding book, yet it should be the foundation of any safe infant-feeding advice: **The full caloric requirement of newborns from birth to one month is 100–120 calories per kilogram body weight per day or an average of 110 calories/kg/day** according to the United Nations and WHO.[30] This provides what's needed to maintain weight and ensure healthy growth, and is equal to 5.5 oz/kg/day or 2.5 oz/lb/day of breast milk or standard formula. The estimated requirement to maintain weight is about 100 kcal/kg/day, which is provided by about 15 ounces a day of mature breast milk or formula for an average 3 kg (6.5 lb) newborn. The average mother produces a total of 2 ounces (60 mL) of colostrum on day 1, 6 ounces (180 mL) on day 2, 12 ounces (360 mL) on day 3, and more than 16 ounces of mature milk each day thereafter.[31] Using this data, the calculated caloric yield of exclusive colostrum feeding provides about 10 percent, 33 percent, and 66 percent of an average 6.5 lb or 3 kg newborn's full caloric requirement on days 1, 2, and 3, respectively (see chart below). Few people know how few calories colostrum provides, because it is never discussed in parent education, and rarely in health professional education.

---

* Note that the calories we are typically familiar with are actually 1,000 calories, or 1 kilocalorie (kcal), scientifically. From this point forward, any reference to "calories" refers to kilocalories.

Calories Provided by Colostrum Relative to the Average Full Requirement of a Term 3 kg Newborn

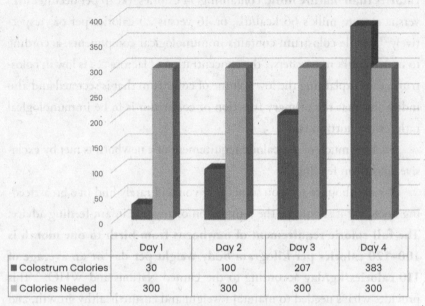

	Day 1	Day 2	Day 3	Day 4
■ Colostrum Calories	30	100	207	383
■ Calories Needed	300	300	300	300

Calculated average caloric yield of exclusive colostrum feeding for an average 3 kg newborn given published colostrum production of healthy postpartum mothers.[32]

Therefore, even though we are taught that newborns receive all that they need from colostrum and that newborn weight loss is from fluid shifts, **exclusively colostrum-fed newborns are in fact losing weight because they are receiving fewer calories than their body requires to maintain their weight**—hence the reason why the ABM refers to this period as a "time-limited duration of underfeeding."[33] They are forced to lose weight as they burn through internal caloric reserves and will eventually experience hunger (and thirst) as they deplete those reserves.

In fact, a 2007 study on exclusively breastfed newborns recognized the period between birth and the onset of lactogenesis II as a period of relative fasting and catabolism (weight loss from burning caloric reserves) marked by low insulin levels and high ketones.[34] This was accompanied by more frequent feedings between days 1 and 2 (now commonly known as "second night syndrome"). If milk came in at day 3, the baby experienced a "refeeding phenomenon," when they went from fasting to a fully fed state, marked by higher insulin levels. Babies who experienced greater than 10 percent weight loss within the five-day study period had more pronounced markers of "starvation" like higher ketones and lower blood sugar.

This relative fasting and fluid restriction was reconfirmed by a 2019 study showing that exclusively colostrum-fed newborns have declining glucose levels and rising ketone and sodium levels until lactogenesis II occurs and they stop losing weight.[35] Another study by the same research group found that when infants who lost greater than 10 percent of their body weight were included, hypoglycemia (glucose < 47 mg/dL) and hypernatremia were common, occurring in about a third of infants.[36]

All together, data on the low caloric intake, weight loss, declining glucose, and rising ketone and sodium levels during the exclusive colostrum feeding period point to one conclusion: exclusively breastfed newborns who are frequently crying and nursing before milk comes are in fact hungry and thirsty. This is also the reason why many babies settle after supplemental feedings; for them, colostrum is not enough to satisfy.

How do the authors of exclusive-breastfeeding guidelines know this period of underfeeding is safe? Yes, the average newborn can survive three days of relative fasting conditions—but at what cost? Further, it has never been determined how long it takes for a newborn to develop *starvation*—brain and vital organ injury caused by insufficient nutrition.[37] Parents and health professionals are commonly taught that newborn infants can be safely sustained on a fraction of their full milk requirement for three days (even up to five),[38] but this claim has *never been proven with any safety data on long-term health outcomes.* The redefinition of adequate feeding for breastfed newborns upon establishment of the exclusive breastfeeding standard—namely, to include weight loss of up to 10 percent, and frequent crying and nursing with lower urine and stool output—stems from a widely promoted cultural bias, not scientific research.

It's also important to remember that, by the WHO's own account, no human population had ever spontaneously relied exclusively on breastfeeding before lactogenesis II, during which infants would be required to subsist on a fraction of their nutritional requirement, before the 1991 launch of the BFHI.[39] Today, exclusive breastfeeding in hospitals has to be vigilantly maintained by a system of parent and health professional training, because our natural instinct is to *feed a crying hungry baby.*

Global data on infant-feeding practices shows that the vast majority of infants, historically, were supplemented to prevent hunger until milk came in, called *prelacteal feeding.* Before the BFHI, health professionals also recognized that these supplemental feeds prevented jaundice, dehydration, and hypoglycemia.[40] Newer research consistently shows the same, that supplemental feedings reduce rates of newborn jaundice, dehydration, weight loss, and hypoglycemia in breastfed newborns[41]—conditions that are among the most common reasons why healthy term newborns are admitted to the hospital today.[42]

MYTH 6:

"If exclusively breastfed newborns produce one wet and dirty diaper each on the first day, two wet and dirty diapers on the second day, and three each on the third day, then they are getting enough milk."

Parents are often told if their exclusively breastfed newborn produces these numbers of wet and dirty diapers, they are getting enough milk. However, since the period before lactogenesis II is a known period of underfeeding, it should be no surprise that they produce fewer wet and dirty diapers compared to when they are fed their full nutritional requirement. The body responds to low milk intake by reducing urine and stool output. The more important question is, are these diaper counts true indicators of adequate feeding?

In fact, diaper counts have been found to be unreliable markers of adequate feeding. A 2008 study showed that exclusively breastfed newborns can produce up to six wet and dirty diapers on day 4 even when they've lost 10 percent of their body weight—an amount health professionals traditionally deem excessive (and an assumption we discuss in the next section).[43]

This suggests that infants will produce wet and dirty diapers from the fluid and meconium (stool) they were born with, regardless of how much nutrition they receive during the first few days, and that diapers cannot tell you if they are getting enough.

MYTH 7:
"Newborn weight loss of up to 10 percent is normal and safe."

While some newborns may tolerate this period of low intake without consequence, we know that those who receive the least colostrum lose the most weight and are at risk for developing medical complications that can impair brain development. So, what percentage of weight loss is unsafe and indicates that brain development may be at risk?

For decades, we believed that up to 10 percent weight loss in exclusively breastfed newborns was normal and safe. In fact, the Newborn Weight Loss Study, which included over 160,000 exclusively breastfed newborns, has found that 10 percent of vaginally delivered EBF newborns and 25 percent of cesarean-delivered newborns lose 10 percent or greater in the first seventy-two hours.[44] But those newborns weren't studied in the years following to determine if the weight loss was in fact safe. The data describes weight loss trends in the first seventy-two hours in infants successfully discharged without requiring special care; it does not tie these numbers to any clinical outcomes in the years after.

There are only two studies on newborn weight loss and neurodevelopmental outcomes. One, from 2002, looked at differences in neurodevelopmental outcomes between newborns admitted with 12 percent or greater weight loss or high sodium levels (a marker of dehydration) compared to newborns without these conditions.[45] However, they relied on parent self-reporting and medical chart review and did not directly measure the infants' development with standardized testing, which is far more accurate. Furthermore, they did this study at twenty-four to thirty-six months of age, when many developmental milestones like full language development, advanced problem solving, and academic proficiency cannot be fully assessed. Hence, the results of this study are of limited use. Similar studies of newborns who develop hypoglycemia, for instance, have shown that neurodevelopment appears equivalent between exposed and nonexposed infants at two years of age.[46] But when those same infants were tested at 4.5 years old, their trajectories diverged, with children who developed newborn hypoglycemia having worse neurodevelopment.[47]

A 2007 study (which, unlike the 2002 research), used standardized developmental tests at age five measured neurodevelopmental outcomes in newborns who developed excessive weight loss of 12 percent or greater. While the authors found no differences in developmental test scores or neurological exams between the excessive weight loss group and the healthy control group, which is encouraging, there *were* other important differences between the two groups. The newborns with excessive weight loss were more likely to fail the fine-motor exam. In addition, parents of these newborns reported higher rates of "shyness," "allergies," and "disability," and were also more likely to report concern about their infant's speech. While there were no differences in speech delay noted by the study psychologist and neurologist, no formal speech evaluations were reported.

Those are all the studies we have on the safety of the 10 percent weight loss threshold: one that used parental reporting and medical records on cognitive development at thirty-six months, and another that indicated worse outcomes in infants with weight loss of 12 percent or more.

Years of research since these studies were conducted have found that complications of insufficient feeding like excessive jaundice, dehydration, high sodium, and low blood sugar can occur *before* 10 percent weight loss, often in exclusively breastfed newborns before lactogenesis II.[48] A 2018 study in which term infants were universally screened for high sodium levels (or hypernatremia, sodium > 145 mEq/L)—a marker for dehydration— found it to be common, occurring in 36.5 percent of exclusively breastfed newborns and 38 percent of mix-fed newborns (possibly those who lost excessive weight from exclusive breastfeeding and needed supplementation), compared to 6 percent of exclusively formula-fed newborns.[49] It also found that hypernatremia could occur at an average of 8.6 percent weight loss and as early as 4.8 percent weight loss. In a 2007 study of newborns admitted for hypernatremia (determined in this research as sodium > 150 mEq/L), more than half were found to have abnormal development at twelve months of age. And a 2021 study of 100 newborns admitted for hypernatremia (≥ 150 mEq/L) found that **more than 45 percent of the 93 newborns who received MRIs had visible brain injury.**[50]

Low blood glucose (or hypoglycemia, glucose < 40 mg/dL) has been shown to occur in 10 percent of exclusively breastfed term newborns and 23 percent of newborns born to first-time mothers.[51] These levels of hypoglycemia have been associated in another study with a 50 percent reduction in passing standardized proficiency tests in math and literacy at ten years of age.[52] A brain imaging study of term infants with symptoms of hypoglycemia and glucose levels of 46 mg/dL or lower showed 94 percent had brain injury on MRI.[53] One case series of newborns developing low blood sugar from poor breastfeeding showed that, despite most (9 of 11) losing less than 10 percent body weight, five of the six MRIs obtained from the infants showed extensive brain injury.[54]

Suboptimal feeding from exclusive breastfeeding is a major risk factor for excessive jaundice (a.k.a. hyperbilirubinemia), according to the AAP.[55] The risk of developing hyperbilirubinemia increases with weight loss of 7–8 percent or greater.[56] In the pre-BFHI era, hyperbilirubinemia occurred in only 6 percent of US term newborns, and was then recognized as strongly associated with breastfeeding;[57] now, it occurs in 30 percent.[58] Hyperbilirubinemia can increase the risk of multiple cognitive and developmental problems, called bilirubin-induced neurological disorder, and a more severe disorder, kernicterus.[59] In a study of jaundiced newborns with bilirubin levels of 20 mg/dL or higher who were followed to thirty years of age, 45 percent had persistent neurobehavior problems; impaired attention and impulsivity; problems with reading, writing, and math; higher rates of remedial or special education; lower rates of completing high school and college; and higher rates of unemployment and alcoholism.[60]

Ultimately, more current studies show that complications of insufficient feeding can and do occur before 10 percent weight loss, and that these complications are associated with high rates of disabilities that can affect a child far into adulthood. Yet this threshold is still commonly regarded as acceptable, even as no studies have confirmed its safety.[61]

MYTH 8:

"Introducing supplemental milk will cause breastfeeding to fail."

Western exclusive-breastfeeding advocates believe that the persistent nursing that occurs by the second day of life is a "biological norm" required to help "bring in the milk," as the stimulation provided by frequent nursing and colostrum removal causes a cascade of hormonal changes that result in the onset of full milk production.[62] In addition, they believe that introduction of supplemental formula reduces the infant's hunger for breast milk, interfering with this necessary cascade. Observational studies do show that mothers who supplement early tend to not breastfeed as long.[63] But do mothers produce less breast milk because they supplement, or do they supplement because they produce less breast milk? These studies cannot say.

What we do know is that breastfeeding mothers in developing countries have long supplemented their newborns until their milk came in. As we saw in chapter one, this practice predates formula. For generations, parents used common sense when breast milk supply was not enough to satisfy their infants, supplementing through wet nursing, animal milk, or sugar water, and did so most commonly in the days immediately after birth. This practice of prelacteal feeding was common in every country—including those with high breastfeeding rates—before the WHO's global push to promote exclusive breastfeeding.

One of the most cited reasons for prelacteal feeding in the developing world is that the initial colostrum is "not enough" to satisfy a newborn infant. Prelacteal feeding, in contrast, was observed to satisfy infants—and prevent jaundice, dehydration, and hypoglycemia until full milk came in.[64] Such supplementation allowed the *infant* to determine how much they received, regardless of how much colostrum their mother produced, thus naturally preventing hunger from insufficient milk intake and the medical complications that might result. The higher quality the substitute, the fewer abnormalities would occur. While feeding potentially contaminated supplements (e.g., raw animal milk) came with risks, it still mitigated the greater risk of starvation from inadequate nutrition. Widely practiced prelacteal feeding during low breast milk production, we can presume, made the modern requirements for monitoring weight loss and bilirubin unnecessary for most healthy newborns.

Prelacteal feeding is commonly viewed by its detractors as counterproductive to promoting breastfeeding, and a barrier to achieving the WHO's exclusive breastfeeding targets.[65] Yet in places where it has been widely practiced, sustained breastfeeding rates were *high*, with most mothers breastfeeding for a median duration of one to two years.

Prelacteal Feeding and Median Duration and Prevalence of Breastfeeding Across the Globe

Country (Survey Years)	Rates of Prelacteal Feeding	Average (Median) Duration of Breastfeeding in Months	Breastfeeding Rates at 1 year/2 years[66]
Bangladesh (1993–94)[67]	90%	>36	95.5%/86.5%
Gambia (2000)[68]	98%	No data	96.8%/53.9%
India (1992–93)[69]	87.9%, 99%	24.4	87.5%/67.5%
Nigeria (1990)	Nearly 100%[70]	19.5	86.4%/42.9%
Pakistan (1990–91)[71]	Nearly 100%	19.9	78.2%/51.7%
South Africa (1998)[72]	47.1% (rest was 57% mix-fed)	16	66.6%/30.4%
Vietnam (1997)[73]	Nearly 100%	16.7	80.2%/23.3%

A 1997 study of infant feeding in Vietnam showed that almost 100 percent of newborns were given prelacteal feeds.[74] Despite this practice, the median duration of breastfeeding was seventeen months, with just a bit more than 80 percent breastfed to one year of age, and nearly a quarter breastfeeding at two years. Fourteen years later, prelacteal feeding in Vietnam was still high, despite one study reporting 73.3 percent of mothers giving prelacteal feeds.[75] Two studies from the 1990s in India showed that 88–99 percent of newborns received prelacteal feeds.[76] The mean duration of breastfeeding in India around that period was twenty-four months.[77] A 1993 study of infant-feeding practices in Bangladesh found that 90 percent of parents gave prelacteal feeds to their newborns, yet Bangladesh's median breastfeeding duration was greater than thirty-six months, with 96 percent breastfeeding at one year and 86.5 percent at two years according to UNICEF data that the same year.[78]

In Hispanic culture, prelacteal feeding is called *las dos*, which means providing both breast and bottle in the days after birth to satisfy hunger, until full milk comes in.[79] Among US Hispanic mothers, 75–80 percent breastfeed, most commonly in combination with formula feeding, and they have higher breastfeeding rates than other racial and ethnic groups.[80] Interestingly, one 2011 study of US breastfeeding mothers showed that Hispanic mothers were 3.81 times more likely to feed both formula and breast milk than white mothers.[81] While combination breastfeeding was associated with shorter duration of breastfeeding among white mothers, no such effect occurred among Hispanic mothers. (One possible explanation is that when a given demographic group believes formula supplementation to be a substandard practice, only mothers in that group who struggle to lactate will use formula—thus producing an association between supplementation and shorter breastfeeding duration.)

While breastfeeding rates have long been high in many parts of the world, according to the WHO's own expert panel, *exclusive* breastfeeding rates were low, due to what many Western breastfeeding researchers deem "misperceptions" among breastfeeding mothers who believe either their colostrum or breast milk supply is insufficient.[82] But who is correct—the researchers, or the mothers? The data on the actual caloric yield of colostrum, and on the rates of delayed lactogenesis II and persistent low milk supply even among mothers motivated to exclusively breastfeed, shows that true low milk supply is common and that the perception of mothers who believe their milk is insufficient are far more correct than we have been led to believe. Furthermore, if supplementation is so detrimental to breastfeeding, then how is it possible that pre-BFHI breastfeeding rates were (and continue to be) so high in so many countries where prelacteal feeding and supplemented breastfeeding were practiced widely? Because it is not. The WHO's own 2017 review of the highest-quality clinical trials found that step 6 of their Ten Steps to Successful Breastfeeding, "Give no food or water other than breast milk, except when medically indicated," **did not** improve rates of breastfeeding after discharge.[83] In fact, the data showed that judicious supplementation *improved* exclusive breastfeeding rates at three months by 20 percent.[84]

There are now *five* randomized controlled trials (the highest standard for primary research) showing that limited supplementation of 10 mL of formula or banked human milk after each breastfeeding at 5 percent or greater than 75th percentile weight loss had no impact on rates of continued breastfeeding (both exclusive and any breastfeeding) at three and six months.[85] Not a single randomized trial has shown that judicious supplementation interferes with sustained breastfeeding. Still, despite data contradicting their current recommendation, the WHO and other supporting organizations continue to back the exclusive breastfeeding rule, and the idea that supplementation compromises breastfeeding continues to be taught to families across the globe.[86]

Supplemented breastfeeding has been practiced for millennia to protect infants from hunger and starvation when exclusive breastfeeding was inadequate to satisfy them. The decision to supplement largely relied on parental observations of infant behavior, *not* laboratory tests or physician diagnoses of "medical indications" for supplementation. This protected the most vulnerable infants whenever milk supply was low, especially in the days after birth. When left to their own devices, parents have a primal need to protect their infants from hunger and respond *appropriately* by providing the safest breast milk substitutes available, because leaving babies hungry *can result in harm.*

When supplementation is practiced along with frequent and effective emptying of breasts, human milk production and direct nursing can be sustained while meeting the full nutritional needs of infants *who need it.* For those whose milk supply increases enough, then supplementation naturally ceases. For those whose supply remains low, supplementation allows their infants to be fully nourished. When supplementation is not stigmatized, as in US Hispanic families, all infants can be protected from malnutrition *without* appreciable declines in breastfeeding rates.[87]

In the same way that prelacteal feeding has been characterized as a "cultural belief," exclusive breastfeeding before lactogenesis II is also a cultural belief, largely of the West—one that comes with significant limitations and risks. Decades of data on insufficient feeding complications during this period now show that the "cultural" phenomenon of prelacteal feeding has a rational, scientifically justified basis in promoting infant survival, health, and development, if done with a safe supplement.

In fact, a world where nearly all babies were exclusively breastfed and thriving has never existed, despite wide promotion of that belief. When safe breast milk substitutes and sanitary feeding vessels were unavailable and breastfeeding was the *only* safe option, bottle-fed infants died in large numbers—an estimated 30 percent.[88] Humans evolved to recognize the signs of persistent hunger and to ameliorate the risks of underfeeding when breast milk was inadequate, and the development of more nutritionally complete breast milk substitutes and more sanitary feeding vessels was an important part of that evolution. Because we prevented infant starvation with supplementation when needed, we as a species have enabled millions of infants to thrive into adulthood who may not have otherwise.

The current messaging around exclusive breastfeeding now invalidates those parental instincts to the detriment of the least-fed infants and the lowest-producing mothers. Now we wait to supplement while babies cry for hours, until they have developed medical complications that put their brains at risk.

While exclusive breastfeeding may be ideal for babies whose mothers have robust milk supplies and who can latch and transfer milk well, it is not ideal for babies who don't. To provide a responsible infant-feeding policy, we must acknowledge the wide variation in breast milk supply, anatomy, and infant nutritional needs, and address those needs in a way that prevents feeding complications and ensures that *all infants thrive*.

WHY DID NATURE CREATE SUCH AN IMPERFECT SYSTEM?

Considering these myths may lead us to ask, "Why would a system evolve that forces a newborn infant to subsist on less than their full fluid and caloric requirement for two to five days until lactogenesis II occurs?" Firstly, nature does not ensure the best outcomes for every child. Nature only requires that enough offspring survive to reproduce and continue the species, selecting against the offspring of those whose physiology (e.g., low milk production) does not ensure their survival. The disadvantaged offspring die or have poor outcomes as a matter of natural selection; only the fittest survive. Therefore, humans have thrived despite our appallingly high historical infant mortality rate (up until the 1900s, an estimated 25–35 percent of infants died before they reached one year of age).[89]

It is important to consider that, at the moment of birth, a mother commonly has been laboring for more than twenty-four hours, using a tremendous amount of energy comparable to strenuous exercise.[90] Laboring mothers are often in a fasting state and may experience significant blood loss. After delivery, mothers may not physically have the excess fluid or calories in their bodies to produce the full milk requirement of a newborn infant (commonly > 500 mL of fluid and 300 calories per day). One hypothesis to explain why mothers produce small volumes of colostrum immediately after delivery is that low production supports the mother's survival; her body prioritizes retaining its remaining calories and fluid, delaying the production of a full milk supply until its reserves have been restored. This relationship is suggested by a study showing that mother–infant pairs who had markers of higher fetal and maternal stress (low umbilical-cord glucose levels and higher maternal exhaustion scores) had higher rates of delayed onset of full milk production.[91] Mothers who experienced higher levels of exhaustion also had lower milk volumes at day 5 after birth. Therefore, the low caloric and fluid content of colostrum may not necessarily be a product of nature's design but merely a *consequence* of the high caloric and fluid demands of labor and the depleted state it causes. This data also suggests that it is not simply the frequency or duration of nursing that determines when milk comes in, or whether supplementation is used, but also the birthing mother's recovery from childbirth.

Ultimately, not all breasts produce sufficient milk, especially in the days after birth, and we evolved as humans to use our intelligence to overcome these limitations by supplementing when necessary. If we consider our parental impulse to feed hungry babies as part of our natural instinct to survive, then it is not nature that is imperfect, but rather the pervasive narrative that exclusive breastfeeding is the *only* healthy way to feed infants and the only way to promote breastfeeding success.

Billions of dollars have been spent over three decades to encourage as many mothers as possible to exclusively breastfeed.[92] Advocates of the EBF policy continue to bemoan that the 44 percent rate of global exclusive breastfeeding at six months is nowhere near the 70 percent target WHO has set for 2030 (a target set with no data on whether EBF is physically possible or safe for 70 percent of mother–infant couplets).[93] Is this a failure of mothers to comply with recommendations? Or is this a failure of health organizations to accept data that a large percentage of mothers may not be able to physically meet this six-month EBF target, and that this near-universally applied recommendation is putting the least-fed infants at risk? The science suggests that it is not the mothers who "misperceive" their own situation but the policy makers who misperceive mothers' and babies' physical and practical realities. By insisting that nearly all mothers can and should exclusively breastfeed, they fail to acknowledge the diversity of biological and social circumstances that define what best infant feeding looks like.

WHAT'S HAPPENING TO MOTHERS, BABIES, AND FAMILIES IN HOSPITALS

Unfortunately, these breastfeeding myths have real-life consequences for infants and their families. Parents and health professionals report that EBF newborns frequently cry and nurse for hours a day in hospitals, a phenomenon dubbed "second night syndrome." For many years, being "fussy at night or constantly feeding for several hours" without "medical indication" *has not* been considered an approved reason for supplementation by the Academy of Breastfeeding Medicine.[94] However, these are commonly the first signs of medical complications like hypoglycemia,[95] hypernatremia,[96] and hyperbilirubinemia[97] from low breast milk intake. The newest 2017 ABM guidelines consider frequent crying and nursing as indications to evaluate the nursing, with no specific guidance on testing for these medical complications in response.[98] According to real-life accounts by clinicians and parents, such policies have resulted in infants developing serious complications after hours to days of constant crying and nursing that were either not recognized or dismissed as signs of distress.[99]

Many of the health professionals who have written to and/or joined the Fed Is Best Foundation have reported having been written up for offering formula when a mother expressed concern that her infant was not getting enough breast milk, because it compromised their hospital's metrics.[100] On the other hand, there are few if any repercussions if an infant who is exclusively breastfeeding is discharged and then returns to the hospital medically ill from insufficient-feeding complications. Some professionals have complied with the guidelines to keep their job despite their ethical objections and have experienced moral injury as they watched infants harmed. Others have left the field of postpartum care altogether because of it.

According to one labor and delivery nurse, Michelle Windsor, who decided to post publicly about her experiences:

I've also worked in the postpartum unit in a different hospital that went all out crazy with the Baby-Friendly [Hospital Initiative]. I have had my share of crying babies and parents. Also, lactation consultants who flat out lie to the parents and tell them their baby isn't hungry. We are telling the parents to ignore their instincts and tell them every mother makes enough for their baby. So, at night, as the moms are sobbing because their baby lost significant weight, is jaundiced and dehydrated, they think they are the only ones not making enough to satisfy their baby. I then have to convince them that every other mother is doing exactly the same thing. All this so that the hospital can get every baby exclusively breastfeeding at discharge so that they may become "Baby-Friendly," which brings in money. When I talk to these parents, they are hearing it for the first time. What I mean is, when I sit them down and literally say that what I'm about to say could get me in trouble or even fired but I don't care. I'm more interested in the health of you and your baby. I then shut the door and talk frankly to them. I honestly stayed as long as I did because I felt that I owed it to my patients to be their advocate.

While breastfeeding initiation rates have indeed risen dramatically with the launch of the BFHI, so have extended and repeated admissions from complications of underfeeding.[101] As a result, exclusive breastfeeding in the days after birth is now the leading risk factor for hospital readmission,[102] and is associated with a two- to elevenfold higher risk for readmission.[103] A study of a large US health system found the leading causes of readmission were feeding problems and jaundice, representing 41 percent and 35 percent of the admissions, respectively.[104] Another study of more than 203,031 infants born in New York State in 2008 found that 4.4 percent (9,010) were readmitted in the first month. Jaundice, dehydration, and feeding problems accounted for 37 percent of the readmissions.

The fact that feeding-related medical complications can occur to exclusively breastfed newborns is *common knowledge* among pediatric health professionals, and yet it is rarely fully described in parenting or breastfeeding literature. This failure to fully inform parents is partially responsible for these complications, yet prominent exclusive breastfeeding advocates and organizations oppose informing parents, stating such a warning would "directly challenge efforts across the US, and around the world, to emphasize the value of exclusive breastfeeding and the risks of unnecessary supplemental feeding."[105] This is a violation of the ethical requirements of health professionals to provide informed consent regarding the benefits *and* risks of medical decisions, including on methods of infant feeding. It would be equivalent to a surgeon leading a patient to accept a surgical procedure by highlighting all its benefits while hiding the risks. No health system in the world—no matter how sophisticated, well staffed, or well funded—can protect every infant from insufficient feeding complications if the parents themselves are not taught how to accurately recognize and prevent them.

Although we can and should continue to support breastfeeding to promote infant health, particularly in places where breastfeeding is the only safe option, we cannot pretend the risks we've just described do not exist. Safe breastfeeding promotion for all infants *is* possible if we can abandon harmful, "abstinence-only" policies that encourage us to wait for a medical emergency before supplementing a hungry infant. The most current studies provide exciting results, because they show we can prevent hospitalizations by supplementing infants before feeding complications occur—*without* compromising a mother's ability to breastfeed.

Historically, parents have always prioritized safe and adequate nutrition over the way their infants are fed. Parents continue to do so, much to the frustration of hospital staff tasked by their superiors to convince those mothers who find their colostrum insufficient that their infants are not hungry, even when these mothers suspect they are. Ultimately, no amount of disinformation or reassurance can convince parents that their babies are getting enough milk when they are not—which is why, after more than forty years, the WHO has failed to accomplish their goals.

The reality is, we have *always* needed both breast milk and supplements to protect the health of all infants. But knowing when supplements are needed is a vital parenting skill left out of most breastfeeding resources—which is why this book is dedicated to teaching every parent how to confidently reach their individual infant-feeding goals while keeping their infants safely and sufficiently fed.

3

Breastfeeding, Formula Feeding, or Both: Is There a Single "Best"?

What is the "best" way to feed your baby? The short and truthful answer is that it depends on you, your body, your baby, their needs, and myriad other factors. In fact, of all the myths we've discussed so far, the idea that there is only *one* best form of feeding for all infants is perhaps the biggest. To dissect this myth, we first must discuss what the research says about breastfeeding and formula feeding, and how a one-size-fits-all message about infant feeding can fail to accurately portray real life—and ultimately fail to serve families who do not fit into a narrow mold.

The global recommendation of exclusive breastfeeding is based on what scientists have found in observational studies for the *average* outcomes of breastfed versus formula-fed infants when measuring different health outcomes like rates of respiratory and gastrointestinal infections, allergic diseases, obesity, diabetes, sudden infant death syndrome (SIDS), and markers of intelligence.[1] However, while some exclusive breastfeeding advocates have suggested these studies indicate that feeding a child human milk *causes* better health outcomes, one limitation of this position is that these studies in fact only show that there is a *correlation* between breastfeeding and better health outcomes. **Correlation does not equal causation, as outcomes from observational studies can be affected by other variables** (called confounding variables). For instance, households with higher income and more educated parents tend to breastfeed more.[2] Since higher household income and education generally improve health outcomes, we can't be sure if it is breastfeeding alone, income and education, or a combination of these factors, that do this. It's possible that access to healthcare, sufficient financial and educational resources, or a healthier parental lifestyle happens to be more common among mothers who end up breastfeeding, and *those* factors are what cause better long-term infant health and intelligence.

The second limitation of making recommendations based on comparisons of average outcomes between breastfed and formula-fed infants is that just because something happens *on average* does not mean it happens *to all*. Population averages showing breastfed infants have better outcomes do not mean that this effect will apply to every single breastfed child. For instance, if a mother does not produce breast milk, then clearly breastfeeding will not produce optimal health outcomes for her child. If a nursing parent has low milk supply, then combination feeding will likely be better than exclusive breastfeeding. Unlike drug trials, where participants who receive the drug being tested each receive the same dose, human milk production varies widely across the population, and therefore exclusive breastfeeding does not result in the same "dose" to each child. Therefore, the outcomes will vary greatly.

We want to arm you with a more balanced perspective on the breast-versus-formula debate by giving you actual numbers on how great a potential effect each feeding option can have on your child's health and developmental outcomes, while being transparent about the limitations of these statistics. We do this so that those who wish to breastfeed, but find they are unable to, understand that there are many other things they can do as parents to ensure the best outcomes for their children.

THE BEST EVIDENCE ON BREASTFEEDING VERSUS FORMULA-FEEDING OUTCOMES

The best available evidence on outcomes of any health-related intervention comes from studies where subjects are randomly selected to either receive an intervention (the "intervention" group) or not (the "control" group). This process of randomization is important because it allows confounding variables that can also affect health outcomes, like socioeconomic status and parental education, to be evenly distributed between the two experimental groups, thereby reducing the effects of these variables and allowing us to see the effect of the intervention alone. The following is not a comprehensive review of breastfeeding research but a discussion of key studies that reduce the effects of these confounding variables.

The best data we have on the effect of breastfeeding promotion comes from the Promotion of Breastfeeding Intervention Trial, or PROBIT, conducted from 1996 to 1997 in Belarus. It is the largest randomized controlled trial ever completed on breastfeeding, with more than 17,000 mother–baby pairs "cluster randomized" to treatment and control groups (meaning that, instead of randomizing the individual infants to the two groups, researchers randomized the assignment by hospital). It randomly assigned sixteen of thirty-one hospitals to receive breastfeeding promotion intervention (the BFHI) and assigned the other fifteen to the nonintervention control group.[3]

The study found that infants in the intervention group did in fact have higher rates of both exclusive and predominant breastfeeding.[4] At three months, infants from the intervention group were seven times more likely to be exclusively breastfed and twice as likely to be predominantly breastfed. Breastfeeding rates at six months were low for both groups, but were higher among infants in the intervention arm, both for exclusive (7.9% versus 0.6%) and predominant breastfeeding (10.6% versus 1.6%). And for the last couple of decades, researchers have been following these infants to see if there are differences in health and intelligence outcomes.

The findings of the study so far were summarized in a 2014 article.[5] Those in the breastfeeding intervention group had lower rates of gastrointestinal infections and atopic eczema in their first year of life, but their rates of developing two or more respiratory tract infections were similar to the control group. There were greater weight and length gains in the first three months of life in the breastfeeding intervention group, but no detectable differences at twelve months. At 6.5 years, children born to the breastfeeding promotion group had a 7.5-point higher verbal IQ, a 2.9-point higher performance IQ, and a 5.9-point higher full-scale IQ, and higher blinded teacher assessments of academic performance, than those in the control group. However, when the children reached sixteen years of age, these differences disappeared.[6] (In a secondary analysis of this study at age sixteen, which corrected for those in the intervention group who did not actually breastfeed—despite being the breastfeeding promotion group—there was a modest 3.5-point higher mean verbal function in the intervention group.) It is also worth noting that the earlier PROBIT IQ studies did not blind the IQ testers to children's birth hospital (and therefore their experimental group), which could have biased results. When the participants were sixteen, computerized intelligence testing was used, which blinded the investigators to their experimental group, thus eliminating this bias. The PROBIT has found no significant differences in rates of childhood asthma, allergic disease, overweight, height, blood pressure, or child behavior.

In July 2018, another analysis of a large number of studies was published that compiled the PROBIT and other published data on breastfeeding and infant health outcomes in a way that made it easier to understand for health professionals and parents.[7] The authors used the data to calculate how many babies would need to be breastfed in order to prevent one infant from developing a disease (a.k.a. the number needed to treat). They provided these numbers while repeating the caveat that the data cannot be used to suggest that breastfeeding had a *causal relationship* to these outcomes (meaning breastfeeding itself prevented the disease)—rather, that what the numbers show is just that these health problems occur less frequently in breastfed infants. The following table details the numbers needed to treat for preventing various childhood diseases.

Number of Babies That Need to Be Breastfed to "Prevent"* One Case of Disease

The fewer babies that need to be breastfed to prevent one case of a disease, the greater the potential effect of breastfeeding on that disease. The more babies that need to be breastfed to prevent one case, the lower the effect.

Disease	Number of Babies
Ear infection before 2 years of age	2–3
Upper respiratory infection (cold)	6–7
Lower respiratory infection (pneumonia)	25
Gastrointestinal (GI) infection	4–30
Necrotizing enterocolitis in preterm baby	25
Hospitalization for GI infection	171
Hospitalization for lower respiratory infection	115
Sudden infant death syndrome	3,500
Acute lymphoblastic leukemia	12,500
For infants with a family history of asthma, eczema, or allergic rhinitis:	
Eczema before 2 years of age	36
Allergic rhinitis (seasonal allergies)	54–70
Asthma	76

The word "prevent" is in quotations because observational data does not prove causation.

Regarding intellectual development, the authors noted that several studies conducted in developed countries have shown that breastfeeding correlates positively with improved IQ. However, studies that compared intelligence outcomes between breastfed and formula-fed *siblings*, and those that considered the effects of maternal IQ, found few to no differences. A 2013 WHO meta-analysis[8] (a study that combines data from all available good-quality studies) found a 2.2-point increase in IQ, and a 2015 meta-analysis[9] found a 1.76-point increase among breastfed infants evaluated during childhood and/or adolescence. The authors suggested a 1.72- to 2.2-point difference in IQ was of "questionable clinical benefit," which means it would be difficult to recognize this IQ difference in real life.

The 2018 review authors found no evidence that breastfeeding protects against:

- food allergies
- dental problems
- hypertension
- type 2 diabetes
- high cholesterol
- height and weight gain
- childhood/adult obesity
- death[10]

Ultimately, the PROBIT and other breastfeeding studies show that breastfeeding has the greatest potential effect on reducing ear infections, gastrointestinal infections, upper and lower respiratory infections, and cases of necrotizing enterocolitis (a life-threatening infection of the small intestines in premature infants) and the related hospitalizations. This is not surprising, given that human milk is known to contain IgA antibodies, which are responsible for protecting the respiratory and gastrointestinal tract from infectious pathogens.[11] Among infants who have family histories, breastfeeding is associated with lower rates of asthma, eczema, and allergic rhinitis (or seasonal allergies).

For leukemia and SIDS, the potential effect is much smaller because these conditions are much rarer. About 33 cases of SIDS occurred per 100,000 babies in the United States in 2019[12] (equal to a 0.003% chance of SIDS). Even with that 64 percent reduction in SIDS risk found among infants breastfed for more than 6 months,[13] that only reduces risk from 0.003 percent to 0.001 percent, a difference that would be difficult to detect for an individual in real life. In other words, it is extremely improbable that you will cause your child to develop leukemia or die from SIDS because you could not or did not want to breastfeed. Even if a definitive causal relationship had been demonstrated (it has not), the effect would be vanishingly small.

Pacifier use in fact has a stronger correlation with lower SIDS rates than breastfeeding. One case of SIDS may be prevented if 2,733 babies used a pacifier, compared to 3,500 babies in the case of breastfeeding (remember, a lower number indicates a more powerful effect).[14] So, if you aren't breastfeeding, you can lower the risk of SIDS with pacifier use instead. Also worth knowing: while avoidance of pacifiers had long been one of the Ten Steps to Successful Breastfeeding,[15] the 2017 WHO expert committee on breastfeeding found insufficient data to support pacifier avoidance and thus dropped the recommendation.[16]

THE POTENTIAL HARMS OF EXCLUSIVE BREASTFEEDING PROMOTION

Modest benefits in disease prevention weren't the only things the 2018 review found, however. It also identified a number of things for which breastfeeding—specifically exclusive breastfeeding—increased the risk.

As the authors of the review reported, "Exclusive breastfeeding at discharge from the hospital is likely the single greatest risk factor for hospital readmission in newborns" and "term infants who are exclusive breastfeeding are more likely to be hospitalized compared to formula-fed or mix-fed infants due to hyperbilirubinemia, dehydration, hypernatremia, and weight loss."[17] EBF late preterm infants (those born at 35–36 weeks, 6 days) are nearly *twice* as likely to be hospitalized due to feeding complications as breastfed term or non-breastfed preterm infants. They calculated that for every seventy-one EBF newborns, one would be readmitted, and that for every thirteen EBF newborns, one would lose more than 10 percent body weight.

The data collected in this review are not the only findings along these lines. Newer data from the Newborn Weight Loss Study[18] showed that EBF newborns are twice as likely to be readmitted as exclusively formula-fed (EFF) newborns, with one requiring readmission for every fifty-one exclusively breastfed newborns.[19] In addition, 13.5 percent of EBF newborns lost excessive weight (≥10%)[20]—which, as we know, increases the risk of excessive jaundice and hypernatremic dehydration—versus 0.09 percent of EFF newborns.[21] That means for every eight newborns exclusively breastfed in the hospital, one will develop excessive weight loss.[22] EBF newborns are also six times more likely to have high sodium dehydration (hypernatremia) than EFF newborns (36.5% vs. 6.25%),[23] resulting in one case for every 3 EBF newborns.[24]

Number of Newborns Needed to Exclusively Breastfeed to Cause One Complication

Complication/Disease	Number of Newborns
Hospital readmission for insufficient feeding complication	51–71
Excessive weight loss (>10%)	8–13
High-sodium dehydration (>145 mEq/L)	3

These numbers may not even capture the full scope of the issue. For every baby that is hospitalized, how many more are "near misses" who were never diagnosed but treated with rescue supplementation? No one knows. However, it would be logical to assume that for less severe (but still serious) complications, supplementation can be given to prevent escalation to the point where hospitalization is necessary.

The problem is not exclusive breastfeeding itself. It is the insistence that breastfeeding *must* be exclusive to be ideal, even when breast milk supply is lower than what can satisfy a baby and meet their full caloric requirement. While breastfeeding usually works well, it does not work perfectly for all families. And while encouraging mothers to trust their bodies may be comforting and even empowering, we must acknowledge the reality that bodily functions sometimes fail to provide the ideal outcomes. So, vulnerable newborns need a better safety net.

So far, out of all the studies published by the PROBIT group, none have studied the *negative* effects of the BFHI policy: the risks of developing feeding complications during EBF, or the number of infants who develop disabilities in the intervention versus the control group. Another major lapse in breastfeeding research: infants whose mothers cannot produce adequate milk are the ones most likely to develop feeding complications while exclusively breastfeeding and ultimately become formula fed. Therefore, it's possible that developing a "medical necessity" for formula can cause some of the negative health outcomes found to occur more frequently in formula-fed babies in observational studies referred to by the AAP and other organizations.[25] To fully assess the benefits and harms of the BFHI policy, investigators also must measure the rates of complications, hospital interventions, readmissions, and childhood disabilities occurring in the two groups.

ESTIMATING THE EFFECT OF BREASTFEEDING BY COMPARING BREASTFED AND FORMULA-FED SIBLINGS

Other studies have used different methods to isolate the health effects of human milk feeding from confounding variables. In a 2014 paper titled "Is Breast Truly Best? Estimating the Effect of Breastfeeding on Long-Term Child Health and Wellbeing in the United States Using Sibling Comparisons,"[26] Colen and Ramey noted that "breastfeeding rates in the U.S. are socially patterned" and are greatly affected by household income and education.[27] So, the authors attempted to measure the effects of breastfeeding amid these other factors by comparing breastfed and formula-fed siblings raised in the same household. They measured eleven variables: body mass index, asthma, obesity, hyperactivity, parental attachment, behavioral compliance, reading comprehension, vocabulary recognition, math ability, memory-based intelligence, and school performance.

When Colen and Ramey compared the breastfed and formula-fed babies, the typical patterns seen in many studies emerged where breastfed babies did better overall than formula-fed babies. However, when they compared breastfed and formula-fed siblings who grew up in the same household, they found no differences on ten of eleven measures. The one difference was in rates of asthma; surprisingly, the breastfed siblings did slightly worse. This suggests that more intangible variables like socioeconomic status, parental education, and ultimately the environment in which the child grows up may be more influential to child health and intelligence than the type of milk an infant receives. A later study found similar results for the health outcomes of infants whose mothers prenatally *intended* to breastfeed, whether or not their infants actually received human milk in the end.[28] The research revealed that infants whose moms had intended to breastfeed but did not had similar rates of ear infections, respiratory syncytial virus infections, and antibiotics usage during infancy compared to infants whose mothers actually breastfed.

These findings can be summed up by the following: *the magic is the mom* (or the parent). The parenting choices, the household environment, and access to health and educational resources likely have much greater influence over a child's health and intelligence than the kind of milk they receive in the first year.*

---

* There is an important caveat about these findings. This data was obtained from a high-income country (HIC) where clean water, sanitation, and formula are more readily accessible than they are in low- and middle-income countries (LMIC). Clearly, in households where safe human milk substitutes are not accessible or affordable, by definition breastfeeding is the best option for infant nutrition because it is the *only* safe option. In such circumstances, it is even more critical to support breastfeeding in a manner that protects the breast milk supply and relationship while ensuring an infant receives the nutrients they need to thrive. However, feeding complications also occur to breastfed babies in LMICs, where excessive jaundice is also a leading cause of newborn hospital admission. Data shows that the severity of disabilities and rates of death from jaundice are higher there than in HICs. Therefore, it is not enough to simply recommend exclusive breastfeeding to mothers in LMICs without fully informing them of the importance of *sufficient* nutrition and the dangers of malnutrition when breastfeeding cannot meet an infant's needs.

SO WHERE DOES THIS LEAVE US?

While referring to comparisons of average outcomes between breastfed and formula-fed infants may make it easier to create a simple, easy-to-remember public health message like "breast is best," this one-size-fits-all message fails to accurately portray the relationships between infant-feeding methods and infant health outcomes at the individual level. Rather than help individual families and health professionals achieve optimal infant nutrition and health for *every* child, promoting such a monolithic message—especially when the conditions of the individual mother and infant don't fit the accepted standard—results in actions that unwittingly expose infants to malnutrition.

What if a mother can't breastfeed exclusively, or at all, or she chooses not to breastfeed for other reasons? Is she ruining her child's chances at having the best health and intelligence? The data says no. There are many factors that are far more influential, like a parent's access and commitment to healthy nutrition, healthy lifestyles, and providing educational opportunities that optimize brain development. More importantly, ensuring adequate nutrition contributes far more to a baby's health outcomes than perhaps anything else you can do as a parent.[29]

Research showing that breastfeeding may confer important health benefits but that parents can obtain similar benefits by making other healthful choices should be celebrated. It means we have options when breastfeeding is not possible or desired.

Increasing recognition of the diversity in lactation potential, social and occupational circumstances, and informed maternal infant-feeding choices has led multiple organizations to amend their position on breastfeeding. These include the UK Royal College of Midwives in 2018[30] and the American College of Obstetricians and Gynecologists in 2016, which stated that although they encourage exclusive breastfeeding for six months, mothers who choose to formula-feed should be supported and respected. Most recently, the United States Department of Agriculture published in their 2020–2025 Dietary Guidelines that they recommend "feeding infants human milk for the first six months, *if possible* [our emphasis]" and that "families may have a number of reasons for not having human milk for their infant," like parental choice, adoption, inability to produce a full milk supply, and occupational pressures.[31] This recognition by major health organizations that breastfeeding is good but not always possible or desirable, that it is important to respect parental choice, and that parents can meet their children's nutritional needs with formula if needed, is a breath of fresh air.

Every parent needs support to reach their feeding goals in a manner that achieves the objective of "best" infant health, whether that's support for breastfeeding, formula feeding, or both. We are lucky to live in an age where safe human milk substitutes are available, so that children who otherwise would have died or had poor health outcomes due to inadequate substitutes don't have to suffer those consequences. It means parents should not feel guilty, inferior, or like they are dooming their children to poor health and life potential if they can't or choose not to meet the expected standard. This gives health professionals and health advocates license to provide infant-feeding advice that is truthful, inclusive, respectful, and supportive of all the circumstances that shape what best infant feeding looks like.

First priority, enjoy your baby. If the feeding method you are using doesn't allow you to do this, change to a feeding method that works for you and your baby. Do not let anyone make you feel bad for your feeding choice. Being a good parent is looking out for both you and your baby.
—Jayme Sue Wright, MSN, RNC-NIC, IBCLC, CCE

4

Safe Infant Feeding: Why Fed Is Best

As parents, we must do whatever it takes to protect our children's safety, health, and future potential. To do so, we must provide safe and *sufficient* feeding to protect every living cell in their bodies. The science of feeding has shown that children who have their nutritional needs met *without compromise or interruption* have the highest potential for future health and cognitive development. Infant nutrition is one of the most important determinants of long-term health, immunity, and cognitive development. So, optimal infant feeding that prevents both acute and chronic malnutrition is an important goal for parents and for global health policy.[1]

According to the World Health Organization:

Children under 3 years of age are vulnerable to poor nutrition; the growth rate during this period is greater than at any other time [. . .] Poor nutrition during the early years leads to profound defects including delayed motor and cognitive development, behavioral problems, deficient social skills, a reduced attention span, learning deficiencies, and lower educational achievement.[2]

Parents who have shared their children's feeding complications with us most often cite *omission of important information and/or miseducation from their breastfeeding resources* as the root cause. Unfortunately, recognizing infant hunger has become more challenging, because many resources that describe infant behavior around the time of birth have normalized signs of hunger and underfeeding to discourage supplementation.

Breastfeeding is a beautiful and healthy way of meeting a newborn's need for milk, comfort, and close contact while providing immune protection. However, insufficient breast milk in the first days after birth, particularly if full milk production (lactogenesis II) is delayed, is common and can result in complications of underfeeding. Does this mean that exclusive breastfeeding is always dangerous, or that parents should exclusively bottle-feed? Absolutely not. But parents *must* be made aware of the possibility of insufficient breast milk feeding. They must be taught its signs and consequences—and the vital importance of supplementation *before* complications occur.

Prior to the modern era, when infant feeding in hospitals was centered on infant satisfaction rather than *exclusive* breastfeeding, both breastfed and formula-fed infants were fed to satisfaction, were rarely hospitalized for jaundice and dehydration, and thus were rarely exposed to conditions that threaten brain development.[3] Today, with comprehensive education, parents can safely and confidently provide their babies with all the benefits of breastfeeding while *also* keeping them safe when supplementation is needed.

In this chapter, we discuss the science of infant feeding and the importance of adequate nutrition for brain development, because understanding the science is essential to knowing how to safely feed your baby. We describe what happens in the body during feeding and fasting, and define the threshold between safe and unsafe feeding, using all the scientific literature that has been published on the matter—because our children depend on it. We also hope to provide health professionals and organizations with the important knowledge they need for improving clinical standards. Knowing how to recognize and prevent feeding complications is the most important way we as parents, health professionals, and health advocates can promote safe feeding and optimal health outcomes for every baby, every time.

Some of the material in this chapter may be upsetting to some, or too technical for others. You may choose to skip ahead to the chapters on *how* to achieve optimal feeding. It may be helpful, however, to review the tables, images, and graphs on pages 77 through 85 that describe well-fed versus underfed babies to help guide your reading.

WHAT A HEALTHY, HYDRATED, AND WELL- FED NEWBORN LOOKS LIKE

A well-fed newborn will appear satisfied after approximately ten to twenty minutes of feeding, whether with breast or bottle, and typically will fall asleep until the next feeding in about 2 to 2.5 hours. (Some slower-feeding newborns may take fifteen to thirty minutes to feed; as long as they are satisfied, this can be normal as well.) This occurs throughout the day and night, as newborns typically do not have the capacity to store fuel in their bodies longer than three hours before needing more. Their sleep interval depends on several factors, including how much milk they receive per feed and how long it takes for their bodies to burn through the fuel, which varies with their individual caloric requirement. Babies who are being adequately fed will appear relaxed, satisfied, and peaceful after they have fed effectively, whether they are drinking breast milk or formula (the calorie content per ounce is roughly the same).

A hydrated baby should have slightly plump skin that bounces back when pushed and does not wrinkle. Their mouths and lips should be moist, not dry, chapped, or cracked, and there should be no pink or red specks (sometimes called "brick dust") in their diapers.

Breastfeeding guidelines commonly say we should expect exclusively breastfed newborns to have one wet and one dirty diaper on day 1, two wet and two dirty diapers on day 2, three of each on day 3, and more than six to eight wet and three or more dirty diapers once full milk production occurs.[4] However, as we saw in chapter two, scientific data actually shows these diaper counts to be *unreliable markers* of adequate feeding until after day 4 of life, as even infants who lose more than 10 percent of their weight can produce more than six wet and dirty diapers in the first four days.[5] Diapers in the first few days are the result of fluids and meconium present in the baby's system from before birth, so even babies who are not eating or drinking anything in the first few days still produce urine and stool as a normal function of their bodies. Newborn babies typically produce dark meconium stools (the stool they are born with) once or twice a day, transitioning from black/dark green to lighter green to yellow as they receive increasing volumes of milk, which clears the meconium out. Once newborn infants are receiving their full milk requirement, they typically produce six to eight wet diapers and three or more dirty diapers a day.

The table that follows provides a summary of the signs of a typical well-fed full-term (or "term") newborn (one born at ≥ 37 weeks gestation) using the *safest, most conservative* criteria of adequate feeding.

Markers of a Well-Fed Newborn Term Baby	
General appearance and signs of satisfaction	• Satisfied with most feedings • Calm and able to sleep for 2–3 hours between most feeds, and wakes easily for the next feed
Weight loss percent	• Losing no more than 7% of their birth weight, per the AAP[6] • Weight loss is at no greater than the 75th percentile on the Newborn Weight Tool (NEWT) (discussed later in this chapter)[7] *Note*: Babies have different tolerances for weight loss depending on the caloric reserve they are born with. EBF newborns lose more weight (average of 5%–7%) because they typically receive less milk than EFF newborns, who lose an average of only 3%–4%. Greater than 7% weight loss increases the risk of excessive jaundice and high sodium dehydration.[8] Some require supplementation earlier despite "average"-appearing weight loss due to having lower reserve.
Physical signs	• Presence of saliva; moist mouth, lips, and tongue • Flat fontanelle (soft spot) • Skin on the hand that bounces back when lightly pinched and does not wrinkle • Minimal yellowing of skin limited to the eyes and face

Markers of a Well-Fed Newborn Term Baby	
Wet and dirty diapers	• Urine that is clear or light yellow and not pink, red, orange, or brown • 6–8 wet and 3–5 soiled diapers/day once full caloric requirements are met *Note*: Research shows diaper counts are unreliable markers of adequate feeding and hydration in EBF newborns in the first four days after birth before lactogenesis II (see chapter two).[9] Exclusively colostrum-fed newborns often produce fewer than three wet and three dirty diapers a day, but these numbers do not guarantee adequate feeding.
Weight gain after milk comes in	• No longer losing weight by 72 hours • 6–8 ounces gained/week (about 1 ounce/day)[10] • Weight is maintained at or around their growth chart percentile, not dropping in comparison • Satisfied with most feeds throughout the day except for 2–3 hours in the early evening, when more frequent feeding and fussiness occurs ("cluster feeding")

Note: EBF = exclusively breastfed; EFF = exclusively formula fed.

If your baby is missing any of these benchmarks, it is important to get them evaluated by your baby's doctor and, if needed, a lactation consultant.

THE CALORIC REQUIREMENT OF NEWBORN INFANTS

Many breastfeeding resources offer advice to parents, but *none* until now have provided the actual number of calories and volume of milk a newborn requires to be adequately fed—which should be the foundation of any infant-feeding resource. Without objective criteria, it's easy to bend the definition of fed versus underfed, which is why such resources fail so many families and why complications of inadequate feeding are so common.

The average *full* caloric requirement of a newborn from birth to 1 month is an average of 110 calories per kilogram of body weight per day to support maintenance of weight plus one ounce per day of growth. The *exact* figures calculated by the Food and Agriculture Organization of the United Nations, the World Health Organization, and the United Nations University (FAO/WHO/UNU) are that the average minimum caloric requirements of newborn infants from 0–1 month are 113 cal/kg/day for boys and 107 cal/kg/day for girls, and these figures change monthly.[11] Your own baby's requirement may be slightly more or less than this average. Following their hunger and satisfaction cues can help you determine their actual need. We recommend that every parent calculate this figure for their own baby when they are born, and recalculate as they grow. See the table on page 153 for how to do this.

Most babies enter a recovery phase after delivery, which commonly results in lower milk intake than their full requirement on the first day, even if offered without limitation. The exact desired amount is unique to each child, depending on their caloric reserve and their body's caloric requirement. That first day, they will usually take somewhere between 15 and 30 mL (0.5–1 oz) per feed every two to three hours if they are fed to satisfaction. This may coincide with the fact that a full-term newborn's stomach has an average volume of 20 mL at birth.[12] As a result of this lower-than-full milk intake observed in the first day or two, most newborns, breastfed *and* formula-fed, lose weight in the first days of life.[13]

Remember, the ABM calls the period before lactogenesis II a "time-limited duration of underfeeding";[14] it's a relative fasting period during which newborns are pulling from caloric and fluid reserves they are born with.[15] Here's the key: newborns are born with different caloric and fluid reserves, depending on their weight, gestational age, and stressors around birth, and therefore have *different tolerances for weight loss*. Infants with minimal reserves may be hungry for more milk and tolerate less weight loss; some with plentiful reserves may be hungry for less. Once they come out of this recovery period, they become hungrier and often need their full milk requirement, whether they are breastfed or formula fed: somewhere between 2 and 3 ounces per feed every 2 to 3 hours. **Ultimately, your newborn is the only one who knows what they are hungry and thirsty for and what they require to be sufficiently fed.**

While breastfeeding is a natural function of a mother's body and usually provides what babies need, breasts, like any organ, can fail to work optimally. And while colostrum is beneficial and rich in antibodies and proteins, the average mother produces small volumes. As discussed in chapter two, **colostrum has fewer calories than a mother's mature milk (16 kcal/oz vs. 20 kcal/oz)**[16] and typically provides fewer calories and less fluid than newborns need to stay fully fed and hydrated.[17] As a result, exclusively colostrum-fed newborns are prone to losing more weight than their supplemented counterparts. These newborns' parents therefore must know when underfeeding reaches dangerous levels.

WHEN UNDERFEEDING BECOMES EXCESSIVE AND UNSAFE

Humans evolved to prevent the serious consequences of persistent hunger by using our instincts to supplement when infants indicate that colostrum or breast milk is not enough. In years past, when we supplemented breastfed infants who showed signs of persistent hunger, severe feeding complications were rare. Unfortunately, since hospitals adopted policies focused on avoiding formula supplementation, these complications are becoming much more common.[18]

As we've established, some newborn weight loss after birth is expected. In the first day or two, newborns take in fewer calories than needed to maintain their weight, even when offered more. However, for some newborns, weight loss from underfeeding can cross a threshold and become unsafe for the brain and other vital organs. This occurs when blood glucose levels drop too low (called **hypoglycemia**), and/or sodium and bilirubin levels rise too high (called **hypernatremia** and **hyperbilirubinemia**, respectively), which we'll discuss in greater detail later.

Currently available science cannot accurately determine where the safe weight-loss threshold lies for an individual baby. This is partly because babies are born with different calorie reserves and therefore have different tolerances for weight loss, plus we have no accurate ways of telling how much reserve a newborn has. Also, not enough research has been done to determine what degree of weight loss reliably results in complications of insufficient feeding severe enough to cause impaired brain development. Data from a large study of weight loss in exclusively breastfed and exclusively formula-fed newborns in the first seventy-two hours have been used to create the Newborn Weight Tool (the NEWT), which is used to define normal newborn weight loss in clinical practice. The NEWT can help detect excessive weight loss earlier than simply applying the previously adopted 10 percent threshold.[19] But the NEWT does not tell us what degree of weight loss results in complications that affect development because it wasn't based on long-term outcomes, just those first seventy-two hours; it only lets us compare babies to similar newborns who were discharged well-appearing.

The current breastfeeding guidelines estimate that those at the highest range of weight loss on the NEWT (≥75th percentile) are at greatest risk. While weight loss greater than the 75th percentile should be considered a reason to fully evaluate an infant for feeding problems, research has shown problems can occur before this threshold.[20] Fortunately, most babies will tell you when their hunger and thirst are becoming excessive—something we'll teach you how to recognize below.

First, however, we should discuss how a newborn's body responds to low calorie and fluid intake and what it does to their cells and vital organs.

Feeding, Fasting, and Dehydration

The laws of feeding and fasting are very simple. We need food and water to live. If our bodies need more food or water, we experience hunger and thirst. Every organism or living creature is born with a certain number of cells, each requiring a minimum number of calories to provide energy for that cell to live. Water is needed to provide the circulation that delivers calories, oxygen, and other substances required for metabolism (the chemical reactions required to maintain life) to our cells. The sum of our cells' energy requirements to carry out activities required to live (e.g., movement, feeding, digestion) is our daily caloric requirement. For an infant, if this minimum requirement is not met by human milk or formula, those calories will come from internal reserves such as fat and muscle. If the minimal fluid requirement is not met by the fluid an infant receives, that fluid will be pulled from reserves of water found in the soft tissues (like the fat under the skin), and the kidneys will reduce urine output.

For newborns, the calories in a full feeding are used within about three hours. If they have not eaten in three hours, or they have not received a full feeding, their bodies must pull calories from internal reserves. Our main source of fuel is glucose from food,[21] but—when fully fed—we also have glucose stored in the liver in a molecule called *glycogen*. We have calories stored as fat, as well. It takes a newborn about twelve hours of fasting from a fully fed state to deplete their glycogen,[22] during which time their body does two things. One, it breaks down protein in muscles and converts it to glucose, a process called *gluconeogenesis* that will eventually slow, in order to preserve vital tissue, causing glucose to decline. Two, it converts fat into ketones, an alternative fuel. Burning glycogen, protein, and fat causes weight loss.

The body does all of this in response to underfeeding in order to maintain constant delivery of calories to the brain and vital organs—because if cells do not receive the minimum number of calories required to live, cell death occurs within minutes.[23] As underfeeding continues, the body develops the complications listed below. If underfeeding is severe enough, it can cause cell injury to the brain and vital organs. Underfeeding becomes unsafe the moment when brain-cell death begins. Brain and vital-organ injury from starvation and dehydration can compromise brain development, long-term health, and survival.[24]

Underfeeding can cause six different complications:

1. **Hypoglycemia**—low blood glucose. Glucose is the main fuel of the body, especially the brain.

2. **Ketosis**—high ketone levels. Ketones are the body's backup fuel during fasting, produced when glucose levels fall too low.

3. **Dehydration**—low body fluid. Dehydration can cause low blood pressure, kidney dysfunction, and abnormal levels of electrolytes (or salts in our body fluid).

4. **Hypernatremia**—high sodium (salt) levels caused by severe dehydration.

5. **Hyperbilirubinemia**—high bilirubin levels, commonly called jaundice (the term for the yellow skin it causes). It commonly results from low milk intake, which can impair elimination of bilirubin, a product of the red blood cells that naturally break down after birth. Severe hyperbilirubinemia is toxic to the brain.

6. **Excessive weight loss**—weight loss greater than what a newborn's brain and vital organs can safely tolerate. When caloric intake is less than what the body needs, the body burns fat and muscle for fuel, which causes weight loss.

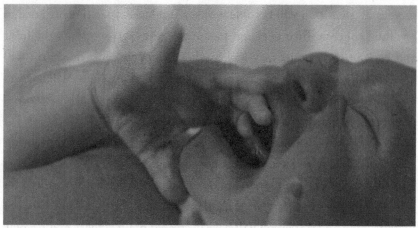

Signs of hunger include fussing and putting hands to the mouth and can progress to persistent, high-pitched crying.

These complications are not the first indications of underfeeding, however. Most term infants will first show signs of persistent hunger.

Hunger in newborns and infants begins with fussiness, accompanied by putting their hands to their mouth and turning their head or rooting as they look for a nipple. If an infant does not receive enough milk, they will persistently fuss or cry, feed for more than thirty minutes—even continuously for hours at a time—and will not sleep more than one to two hours before fussing for the next feed. If a mother does not have sufficient milk at the breast or is not transferring milk sufficiently, the infant's fussiness will progress to constant, high-pitched crying—even with frequent breastfeeding. Babies may latch and unlatch repeatedly as they look for a source of milk to satisfy their hunger. If a persistently hungry baby exhibiting this behavior does not receive adequate milk, then, as they lose weight, they will develop any combination of high blood sodium levels from low body fluid (dehydration), high bilirubin, low glucose, and high ketone levels (which, if underfeeding continues, eventually become depleted).

High bilirubin manifests as jaundice, a yellowing of the whites of the eyes and the skin, starting from the head and progressing downward to the chest, arms, and legs as bilirubin levels rise. Dehydrated newborns have fewer wet diapers; dark urine and/or pink or red dust in diapers; minimal or sticky saliva in their mouths; and dry, cracked lips.[25] As dehydration progresses, their skin will become wrinkly and loose when pinched, due to low fluid content. Their eyes and fontanelles (the "soft spots" on the front and back of their head) may look sunken. Hypoglycemic newborns will appear shaky and have persistent or high-pitched crying. Some will have no symptoms at all. Severe hypoglycemia can result in blank staring, seizures, poor feeding, lethargy, and abnormal breathing.

If a newborn continues to receive less than their full milk requirement, eventually glucose and ketones become depleted, and the amount of energy available to fuel the brain and vital organs dips below what is required for cells to function and survive. An infant crossing the threshold between underfeeding and starvation will have decreased brain activity and become weak due to reduced fuel in their system. They will not have the energy to sustain latch and will become excessively sleepy or lethargic, not waking spontaneously every three hours for feeds. Low heart rate, body temperature, and breathing, as well as seizures, can result. These are *late* danger signs of a severely underfed infant.

Signs of Poor Feeding in Newborns[26]	
Early Stages	**Late Stages**
Signs of Stress from Poor Feeding	*Signs of Brain Dysfunction*
• Excessive hunger signs—frequent, prolonged feeding throughout the day or night (more often than every 2 hours, longer than 30 minutes per feed)*	• Lethargy, listlessness • Limpness, low muscle tone • Poor suck or refusal to feed • Hypothermia or low body temperature
• High-pitched crying; a scream-like cry • Irritability • Tremors, jitteriness • Fast breathing • Sweating • Pallor (pale skin) • Tachycardia (high heart rate) • Jaundice (yellow skin that starts from the eyes and face and progresses down the body) • Cracked, dry lips; sticky or no saliva • Red or pink dust in diapers • No wet diapers for 6 hours	• Sunken fontanelles (soft spot on the head) • Seizures or muscle jerking • Abnormal arching of the baby's back • Irregular or cessation of breathing • Slow heart rate • Cyanosis (blue skin from reduced breathing) • Blank staring • Coma

Note: Cluster feeding should only occur for no more than 3 hours per day, and only after milk has come in.

Any signs of poor feeding should prompt you to ask your health professionals for a full evaluation of breastfeeding latch and technique; a weight check to calculate percentage weight loss and NEWT percentile; weighted feeds; manual expression or pumping to assess milk supply; and testing for blood glucose, sodium, and bilirubin levels (see table below). Abnormal blood glucose, sodium, and/or bilirubin levels or excessive weight loss may require medical interventions (like oral or IV dextrose, IV fluids, or photo-therapy, respectively) to correct. But they can also be corrected with sup-plementation. If the parent's milk supply meets the full caloric requirement of the newborn, then expressed breast milk can be fed by bottle, syringe, or another preferred method. Otherwise, infant formula or banked donor milk can be used, especially if the mother's full milk supply is not in.

Blood Levels That May Indicate Poor Feeding and Dehydration	
Blood glucose (sugar) levels	<50 mg/dL in the first 48 hours and <60 mg/dL beyond 48 hours[27]
Blood sodium levels (a reliable marker of dehydration[28])	>145 mEq/L
Blood bilirubin levels	>13.5 mg/dL • 13.5–19 mg/dL is associated with increased risk for developmental delay and bilirubin-induced neurological disorder[29] • > 19 mg/dL correlates with a rise in blood markers of brain injury,[30] and higher rates of childhood and adult neurodevelopmental problems[31]

It is very common to hear frantically crying babies on the mother–baby units because they are hungry and are not satisfied from breastfeeding. This happens every single shift I work. Mothers are told their babies have "the second night syndrome" and that this is normal newborn behavior. At times, I will admit exclusively breast-fed babies [to the NICU] for hypoglycemia after failed supplemen-tal feeding trials. These babies failed to get adequate calories and fluid at the breast. Often, they should have been admitted much sooner, but the drive is to keep them with their mother and nursing. These babies have suffered hours of hypoglycemia, which causes brain injury every minute it is left untreated. I also admit babies for phototherapy to treat excessive jaundice who have no risk factors beyond excessive weight loss and exclusive breastfeeding. Weight loss at 24–48 hours of 5–9 percent is common for at least 70 percent of our exclusively breastfed babies.[32]

—Debra, neonatal nurse practitioner at a Baby-Friendly Hospital

HYPOGLYCEMIA

Glucose is the most important chemical that provides calories to our cells. It is the primary fuel of the brain, an organ that is very sensitive to glucose deprivation, especially in newborns.[33] Our bodies respond to declines in glucose and fluid reserves by signaling hunger and thirst—something babies communicate by fussing and crying until they are satisfied. According to the Pediatric Endocrine Society (PES), **the sensation of stress and hunger is stimulated by a blood glucose of less than 55 mg/dL.**[34] Temporary declines in brain function through direct measurement of newborn brain activity occur at glucose levels of 47 mg/dL or less.[35] Low blood glucose, or **hypoglycemia**, ultimately results from one or more of the following: receiving too few calories, having insufficient caloric reserve, having a higher caloric requirement, or having insulin levels that are too high (as in babies with diabetic mothers). Once a mother's milk comes in and/or a baby is receiving their full 110 cal/kg/day requirement, normal glucose levels are then maintained.

According to the PES, "Because the brain has only a few minutes' worth of stored fuel reserves . . . interruption of glucose delivery can have devastating consequences. Whereas recovery from brief periods of hypoglycemia is usually complete, severe and prolonged hypoglycemia can cause permanent brain injury."[36] This irreversible consequence is the reason why ensuring an infant is adequately fed is one of the most important requirements of safe and optimal newborn care.

As we discussed, when glucose levels are low, the body can use ketones as an alternative fuel to protect the brain—but *only* if ketone levels are high enough. It is unclear how long an infant can subsist on ketones and what levels are sufficient to prevent brain injury, because no studies have been done. Sometimes, glucose and ketone levels are too low to protect the brain. Some newborns are considered "at risk" for brain-threatening hypoglycemia due to impaired ketone production and are therefore monitored with glucose checks after birth (e.g., premature infants, those small or large for their gestational age, and infants of diabetic mothers).[37] Note, however, that it is also possible for healthy term breastfed newborns to develop unsafe low blood sugar from inadequate feeding—yet they are currently not monitored until they develop symptoms. **Unfortunately, research suggests that if we wait for symptoms of hypoglycemia to occur in healthy newborns instead of preemptively monitoring for it, by the time brain injury becomes obvious, hypoglycemia symptoms (low blood sugar or glucose < 47 mg/dL) already may have occurred.[38]**

Correction of the hypoglycemia would only limit further injury and disability; it would not necessarily reverse it. An MRI study of previously healthy term newborns with hypoglycemia symptoms (glucose < 47 mg/dL) showed that 94 percent had evidence of brain injury.[39] Follow-up on these infants was limited to eighteen months, yet the researchers found 65 percent of them already showed developmental impairment.

While a few minutes of hypoglycemia, corrected quickly, may have no effect, if we wait for symptoms to occur before testing for it, an infant already may have been hypoglycemic for hours, resulting in irreversible declines in cognitive ability that could have been prevented with adequate feeding. We point this out because in a study of medico-legal cases of hypoglycemia resulting in brain injury, the most common presenting sign was "abnormal feeding behavior."[41] Among these behaviors were "not waking for feeds, not latching at the breast, not sucking effectively, appearing unsettled and demanding very frequent feeds." Most of these cases were breastfed newborns, and their parents' concerns regarding inadequate feeding were often dismissed by health professionals.

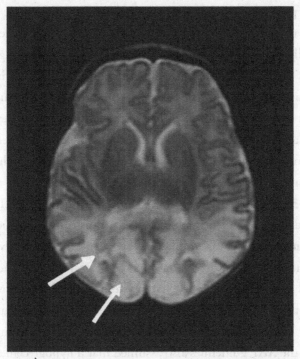

Hypoglycemic brain injury. The image shows normal brain tissue in the top half of the image of the brain. The white areas in the bottom half represent injured tissue caused by severe hypoglycemia.[40]

66

My child went through this trauma. He was born healthy and was fed continuously . . . for the first two days. He was irritable and was always rooting in spite of being fed continuously. Twenty-four hours later he became unresponsive and was taken to NICU, where they stated that his blood sugar dropped to 0. The baby didn't get any milk from me at all. He had brain injury because of this. One-third of his brain got affected due to severe dehydration and hypoglycemia.

—Parent who asked to remain anonymous

The threshold at which hypoglycemia causes brain injury has been hotly debated for decades.[42] Since we know that energy deprivation to the brain can progress to injury within minutes, physicians have sought to determine the lowest safe glucose level. The original safe glucose threshold was initially established using two 1988 studies: one showing that glucose levels below 47 mg/dL caused transient declines in newborn brain activity,[43] and another showing that premature infants with glucose levels below this had higher rates of impaired mental and motor developmental scores at eighteen months of age.[44] Unfortunately, the definition of hypoglycemia was subsequently lowered in response to data that glucose levels commonly declined in the transitional first three hours after birth to around 30 mg/dL.[45] As a result, the authors of the 2011 AAP hypoglycemia guidelines assumed that since these transiently low glucose levels were so common, they were unlikely to be harmful to brain development. The AAP thus redefined normal as glucose of 25 mg/dL in the first four hours, and 35 mg/dL from four to twenty-four hours, for monitored at-risk infants with no symptoms of hypoglycemia.[46] For babies that *do* show symptoms, hypoglycemia was defined as glucose of less 40 mg/dL. The authors of the AAP guidelines also assumed that if hypoglycemia occurred without symptoms, it was unlikely to be harmful to brain development. Unfortunately, there was little data at the time to determine whether these assumptions were correct.

Newer data suggests these transitional lower thresholds may not be as normal or safe as we once believed. Long-term outcomes of transitional hypoglycemia without symptoms have been reviewed in a 2015 study looking at rates of passing the literacy and math proficiency tests at ten years of age.[47] Newborns were universally screened for hypoglycemia in the first three hours; later testing showed that infants exposed to glucose levels of less than 45 mg/dL were 38 percent less likely to pass the literacy test compared to nonhypoglycemic newborns. The outcomes were worse for newborns with glucose less than 40 mg/dL, which were associated with about 50 percent lower rates of passing both the literacy and math proficiency tests. These relationships were found after accounting for demographic and socioeconomic factors and even when researchers excluded premature and high-risk infants from analysis.

A 2018 Swedish population study of more than 100,000 healthy new-borns who developed hypoglycemia (defined as glucose < 40 mg/dL) had similar findings. Hypoglycemic infants had more than double the risk of developmental delay, almost double the risk for motor delay, and almost tri-ple the risk of cognitive delay.[48] Infants experiencing hypoglycemia during the transitional period (i.e., at < 6 hours old) were at higher risk for motor, cognitive, and developmental delay than those with later hypoglycemia (at > 6 hours old).

Last, in a robust 2017 study using continuous glucose monitoring (a device that measures glucose levels constantly without repeated blood draws and can detect hypoglycemia *without* symptoms) showed that at-risk newborns who develop hypoglycemia below 47 mg/dL *at any time*—even without symptoms—had more than double the risk of impaired exec-utive function (problem-solving ability) and more than triple the risk of impaired visual–motor function (coordination of movements using vision) by 4.5 years of age. Contrary to what health professionals have assumed for decades, newborns exposed to hypoglycemia *without symptoms* had *worse* outcomes and were *four times* more likely to have low executive function than those with symptoms.[49]

The consequences of hypoglycemia are serious and irreversible, and some of the worst outcomes published in the medical literature have occurred in previously healthy term breastfed newborns who developed symptoms of severe hypoglycemia.[50] According to Dr. Jane Harding, a leading newborn-hypoglycemia researcher, "Most episodes of hypoglyce-mia occur in the first 48 [hours] . . . when breastfeeding is being established and the supply of milk is low."[51] She has "cautioned against any reduction in operational [glucose] thresholds because the overall rate of [brain devel-opmental] impairment was high and . . . episodes of low glucose . . . were very common." In her study of healthy term newborns (who, remember, are currently not monitored for hypoglycemia unless they have symptoms), the majority of whom were exclusively breastfed, blood glucose levels of less than 47 mg/dL were common, occurring in 39 percent[52] (in at-risk new-borns, they occur in 58.7%[53]). These findings contradict what has long been believed by health professionals: that (1) hypoglycemia without symptoms and "transitional" glucose levels between 25 and 45 mg/dL in the first four to twenty-four hours do not cause brain injury or impaired brain development; and (2) that healthy, term, exclusively breastfed babies are not at risk for brain injury from hypoglycemia.[54]

Given this recent data, **the safest glucose levels for a newborn baby are greater than 50 mg/dL for the first forty-eight hours after birth and greater than 60 mg/dL after forty-eight hours**, a threshold endorsed by the PES as the most protective threshold for the newborn brain.[55] Currently, only newborns considered at risk are screened for hypoglycemia. Healthy, term, breastfed newborns are not, until symptoms occur—despite data that now shows they are also at risk.[56]

Therefore, if your infant is crying and nursing frequently in the first days of life and you suspect that they are not getting adequately fed, we suggest requesting a glucose check from your nurse or doctor if your preference is to continue exclusively breastfeeding. If your baby's glucose is below 50 mg/dL in the first forty-eight hours or 60 mg/dL thereafter, and you have already fed all the human milk you can, then supplementation with banked donor milk or formula to satisfaction is needed to stabilize glucose levels. If an infant is not alert enough to feed by mouth, then IV glucose may be needed.

Some hospitals have adopted giving oral glucose (dextrose) to correct glucose levels while avoiding more invasive IV glucose correction and formula supplementation. But oral dextrose is only helpful in *temporarily* correcting hypoglycemia and is less effective than formula or banked donor milk.[57] Similarly, expressed colostrum is inadequate to correct hypoglycemia given its limited caloric content.[58] Ultimately, there is no replacement for providing an infant their full caloric requirement with nutrition that provides carbohydrates, protein, and fat to stabilize glucose levels.

Disturbingly, research also tells us that the period between discharge and the first doctor's visit is also the highest-risk period for exclusively breastfed newborns. A study has found that infant glucose levels reach their lowest point forty-eight to fifty-nine hours after birth, when most healthy term newborns are discharged from the hospital.[59] If milk does not come in to provide the full caloric requirement, the baby's glucose will continue to decline. This means that during a critical period, when exclusively breast-fed newborns are relying on their mother's full milk supply to come in to prevent further declines in blood glucose, most infants are home where there are *no* health professionals monitoring. Meanwhile, many birthing parents—22 percent of all mothers and up to 44 percent of first-time mothers—will experience delays in milk coming in.[60] If parents aren't taught the signs of hypoglycemia and when it is necessary to supplement, and milk does not come in on time, then their infants will be at risk for developing injurious levels of hypoglycemia.[61]

DEHYDRATION AND HIGH SODIUM LEVELS

A second concern stemming from inadequate milk intake is dehydration, or low body fluid, which is another source of weight loss. Fluid is important for normal cell function and circulation, which delivers oxygen and nutrients to our brain and vital organs. The normal fluid requirement of a newborn is approximately 100 mL/kg/day.[62]

One severe consequence of dehydration is called *hypernatremia,* or high sodium, which results when body fluid is so low that the blood sodium becomes concentrated. Hypernatremia is defined as a sodium level above 145 mEq/L, and it is an indication for medically necessary supplementation. Levels above this number rarely occur when fluids are readily accessible, because a rising sodium level causes thirst and prompts a person to immediately seek fluids. Newborn infants who are developing hypernatremia experience thirst, which will cause them to cry persistently to obtain more fluid through milk.

According to a systematic review on breastfeeding-related hypernatremia, signs of hypernatremic newborns are "poor feeding, poor hydration state, jaundice, excessive body temperature, irritability or lethargy, decreased urine output, and epileptic seizures." Hypernatremia can result in brain injury, organ injury, and increased risk of death.[63] Cessation of breathing, abnormally slow heart rate, seizures, and/or lethargy were frequently present. Of the 1,074 hypernatremia cases reviewed, 64 percent resulted in acute kidney injury, 5 percent caused liver injury; and 6 percent led to brain injury. Death from brain injury occurred in a bit more than 2 percent of newborns.[64]

Hypernatremia-induced brain injury can cause long-term disabilities in survivors. In one study of hypernatremic newborns (≥150 mEq/L), an astounding 45.2 percent had brain injury on MRI.[65] Another study found that among infants with hypernatremia above 150 mEq/L, 50 percent had evidence of developmental delay by one year of age.[66] Yet another found rates of developmental delay of 21 percent at twelve months, 19 percent at eighteen months, and 12 percent at twenty-four months.[67] The largest follow-up study, done to thirty-six months, found that 17.5 percent of hypernatremic infants had developmental impairments.[68] While research showing that rates of developmental delay steadily decline over time may seem reassuring, it's important to remember that developmental studies at twenty-four to thirty-six months provide limited data on long-term outcomes. Similar research on hypoglycemia shows that while development may appear similar between affected and unaffected newborns at two years, outcomes diverge at 4.5 years when more advanced cognitive function emerges.[69] Unfortunately, from cases we have reviewed informally and that Christie has reviewed formally as an expert witness in lawsuits, some of the most severe disabilities have occurred in hypernatremic newborns.

Prior to the adoption of BFHI policies, hypernatremia was rare. But multiple articles have noted that rates of hypernatremic dehydration have been increasing since the policies were introduced, and that it primarily occurs in breastfed newborns who do not get adequate milk.[70] Since there have been no universally adopted standards for hypernatremia screening, how often it occurs and at what percentage weight loss has been unclear. Studies from the 1990s and early 2000s found hypernatremia occurred in less than 1 percent of newborns—but sodium levels were not checked in all newborns (as is still the case today), only in the sickest, most dehydrated babies.[71] Therefore, these studies likely missed less severe cases, thereby underestimating the true incidence.

However, a 2019 study has found that hypernatremia is in fact common among breastfed newborns.[72] Term newborns who were born healthy, 81 percent of whom were breastfed, were universally screened for hypernatremic dehydration (>145 mEq/L). Researchers found that hypernatremia occurred among 36.5 percent of exclusively breastfed newborns and 38 percent of mix-fed newborns (those who likely began as breastfed and developed a need for supplementation due to excessive weight loss). In contrast, 6.25 percent of formula-fed newborns developed hypernatremia. The researchers also found that hypernatremia occurred at lower weight loss thresholds than previously estimated and that the mean (average) weight loss for hypernatremic newborns was 8.6 percent, compared to 6 percent for those with typical sodium levels. Furthermore, for male infants delivered by cesarean by mothers with higher education levels, the threshold for developing hypernatremia was shown to be as low as 4.8 percent weight loss. This provides evidence that complications of underfeeding can and do occur below the 10 percent weight loss threshold that clinicians accepted as normal for decades, and that far more breastfed newborns need supplementation before that threshold is reached. It also suggests that avoiding supplementation until 10 percent weight loss occurs may be putting many infants at risk.

Another important lesson from these studies is that it is not the type of milk that determines whether babies become dehydrated (as well as hypoglycemic), but the *amount* of milk they receive. Formula-fed newborns, too, can develop hypernatremia if they are inadequately fed or the formula is prepared improperly. This provides further evidence of a sound evolutionary reason why families across the globe supplement persistently hungry breastfed newborns before milk comes in, and that the current method of promoting breastfeeding by avoiding supplementation is causing unacceptably high rates of complications that can have long-term consequences.

EXCESSIVE JAUNDICE

Jaundice is common among newborns, occurring in more than 80 percent. Most of these cases are benign.[73] Excessive jaundice, or hyperbilirubinemia, however, often requires hospital intervention like phototherapy to prevent even higher bilirubin that can cause brain injury. It is the most common cause of extended and repeat hospital admission of healthy term newborns in the US and globally.[74] The most common form of hyperbilirubinemia, previously called *breastfeeding jaundice* or *starvation jaundice*, is now euphemistically called *suboptimal feeding jaundice*, and is primarily caused by inadequate milk intake in breastfed newborns. Multiple studies have confirmed that excessive weight loss from suboptimal milk intake is correlated with higher rates of jaundice and that weight loss above 7–8 percent increases the risk.[75]

According to the Academy of Breastfeeding Medicine:[76]

> In newborns, breastfeeding difficulties or a delay in the onset of secretory activation (lactogenesis II) may result in lower caloric intake, which may lead to an increase in enterohepatic circulation [return of bilirubin from the GI tract to the liver] and the development of hyperbilirubinemia. Because formula-fed infants are typically given volumes of milk much greater than physiologically normal (27 mL formula per feeding or about 150 mL/day), during that same period, it is uncommon for them to become jaundiced.

As mentioned, jaundice is caused by bilirubin, a product of the normal breakdown of fetal red blood cells after birth. Bilirubin is eliminated through digestion. The more milk a baby gets, the more bilirubin is removed. Infants who receive inadequate milk are more likely to have bilirubin accumulate in the blood. Since exclusively colostrum-fed newborns are typically receiving less than their full caloric requirement until the milk comes in, higher bilirubin levels are common among them during those first few days.

The AAP lists several risk factors for excessive jaundice, including pre-maturity, family history of newborn jaundice, scalp bruising during delivery, East Asian heritage, and, most commonly, exclusive breastfeeding if feeding is suboptimal.[77] Prior to the adoption of the BFHI, only about 6 percent of newborns developed hyperbilirubinemia.[78] With increased adherence to the BFHI policy of avoiding supplementation in breastfed newborns, rates of hyperbilirubinemia in the US have risen to 30 percent of term newborns, with only 2 percent occurring as a result of jaundice arising from faster breakdown of red blood cells for reasons besides insufficient feeding.[79]

Excessive jaundice in newborns can cause acute bilirubin encephalopa-thy (ABE), or abnormal brain function. ABE causes low muscle tone; high-pitched/scream-like crying; varying degrees of drowsiness; poor feeding; head, neck, and back extension; upward gaze; and a blank, staring, mask-like face. Severe cases can cause respiratory failure, coma, seizures, and, rarely, death.

Survivors of ABE can develop a chronic disability called **kernicterus,**[80] a dreaded complication that causes severe brain injury, cerebral palsy, intel-lectual impairment, and hearing loss, with children often becoming wheel-chair users. Kernicterus is caused by extreme hyperbilirubinemia (>25–35 mg/dL). The Joint Commission (2001), the CDC, and the AAP have all noted that reported cases of kernicterus have risen since the early 1990s—around the time of the adoption of the BFHI.[81] These organizations also noted that breastfeeding is an important risk factor for severe hyperbili-rubinemia, and that it occurs in otherwise-healthy newborns who are not receiving adequate nutrition and hydration through breastfeeding. Despite this, few parents have been informed about these risks of inadequate feeding and how they can be prevented with supplementation when breastfeeding is insufficient, which is why hospitalizations for suboptimal-feeding jaundice are the leading causes of term newborn admissions[82] and why kernicterus continues to occur.

What bilirubin level is considered safe? Current AAP guidelines don't provide a specific threshold at which injury begins to occur. Rather, the guidelines are geared primarily toward preventing the more severe complication of kernicterus using a treatment called phototherapy, a blue-green light that converts bilirubin to a form that can be eliminated through the urine. Phototherapy treatment is warranted at varying bilirubin levels, depending on how many hours old a newborn is and their risk factors. More severe cases of hyperbilirubinemia require exchange transfusion, which involves giving blood products to the baby.[83] The AAP acknowledges these guidelines are based on "expert opinion rather than strong evidence."[84]

Note that several large studies suggest that bilirubin levels below the threshold for phototherapy treatment are still associated with increased risk of developmental delay and disability. One large population study of more than 50,000 newborns showed that moderate hyperbilirubinemia with bilirubin levels between 13.5 and 19 mg/dL increased the risk of developmental delay by 60 percent.[85] Multiple studies show that bilirubin levels above 19–20 mg/dL increase the risk of developmental disabilities.[86] Studies looking at blood markers of brain injury in newborns also show a significant increase in these markers at bilirubin levels around 19–20 mg/dL.[87] In fact, one study that followed jaundiced newborns to the age of thirty found that, among the infants who had bilirubin levels of 20 mg/dL or greater, an astonishing 45 percent had some form of neurological or behavioral challenge, including experiencing problems with reading, writing, and math; problems with attention, hyperactivity, and/or impulsivity; inability to graduate high school and college; lower adult life satisfaction scores; and higher rates of alcoholism.[88] They were 4.7 times more likely to have neurodevelopmental problems compared to the nonjaundiced group, which had rates of impairments closer to those found in the general population.

Unfortunately, the AAP guidelines don't fully address these moderate levels of hyperbilirubinemia. According to the AAP, "Phototherapy should not be used solely with a goal of preventing subtle adverse neurodevelopmental findings, because the literature linking subtle abnormalities with bilirubin is conflicting; there is no evidence that phototherapy improves or prevents any of these outcomes."[89] But this is unlikely to feel like an acceptable risk to parents, who must deal with these "subtle adverse findings" and who rightfully expect *zero* risk of brain impairment from their infants' clinical guidelines.

While using phototherapy to treat these moderate bilirubin levels (13.5–20 mg/dL, for instance) may be excessive or unnecessary, we should not forget that bilirubin levels can *also* be reduced by ensuring adequate feeding. If an infant is approaching bilirubin levels associated with developmental delay and is receiving less than their full milk requirement through breastfeeding alone, then supplementation to satisfaction with banked donor milk or formula can prevent further increases in bilirubin.[90]

We see this clearly in a 2018 US study on jaundiced newborns. The study mainly looked at the effects of treating jaundiced newborns with phototherapy right before they reached the threshold for phototherapy, which reduced readmission for jaundice fourfold.[91] But researchers also found that infants who received formula also were less likely to get readmitted for phototherapy. Those who received zero to two formula feedings per day were 40 percent less likely to get readmitted; those who got six or more were 75 percent less likely. Though the study didn't include banked human milk supplementation, other research suggests that adequate feeding—whether with formula or breast milk, or both—reduces jaundice. If supplementation fails to adequately reduce bilirubin, then phototherapy can be used.

A similar clinical trial found that early supplementation with 10 mL/kg of formula after each nursing session for infants who lose more than 4.5 percent of their body weight within twenty-four hours or in the three days after birth significantly reduced the risk of developing hyperbilirubinemia.[92] Interestingly, researchers found that waiting to supplement until 7–8 percent was lost did *not* reduce cases of hyperbilirubinemia. As with hypernatremia, rates of hyperbilirubinemia increase with weight loss above 7–8 percent. With hyperbilirubinemia, fed is best.

EXCESSIVE WEIGHT LOSS

Weight loss is the measure of infant health that parents are often most familiar with. All newborns are weighed at birth during their hospital stay and once daily until discharge. Weight continues to be monitored at every doctor appointment and is assigned a percentile based on the Newborn Weight

Tool (NEWT) for the first three days after birth, and on the NEWT "First 30 Days" chart thereafter (newbornweight.org). But where do the numbers on these charts come from? What data is it based on?

In the case of the NEWT, the numbers come from a large study published in 2015 called the Newborn Weight Loss Study, which measured the weight loss of more than 160,000 healthy, term, exclusively breastfed (EBF) newborns and more than 7,000 healthy, term, exclusively formula-fed (EFF) newborns who were successfully discharged from the hospital without need for specialty or intensive care. The study found that for formula-fed infants, the average total weight loss is typically 3–4 percent, with a maximum weight loss of 7–8 percent of their birth weight.[93] For exclusively breastfed newborns, the average total weight loss is 7–8 percent, with 10 percent of vaginally delivered and 25 percent of cesarean-delivered babies losing excessive weight of greater than 10 percent.[94] And it used the data collected to create four graphs that show the distribution of weight loss experienced by four categories of newborns during the first seventy-two hours. The four categories of newborns are: (1) EBF vaginally delivered, (2) EBF cesarean-delivered, (3) EFF vaginally delivered, and (4) EFF cesarean-delivered. These graphs are the basis of the Newborn Weight Tool (NEWT), which allows clinicians to determine how an individual newborn's weight loss compares to similar newborns at any time within this period and identifies infants who are losing excessive weight earlier than with the previously used 10 percent weight loss standard.

The NEWT, which is endorsed by the ABM's supplementation guidelines, is now replacing the outdated and unsafe 10 percent weight-loss rule as the standard of care for determining whether an infant requires more intensive breastfeeding management and/or supplemental milk. Intervention is based on whether newborns show weight loss greater than the 75th percentile on the graphs on pages 101 and 102;[95] for instance, a weight loss of 7 percent within the first twenty-four hours is higher than occurs in 95 percent of newborn infants, thus indicating a greater risk of feeding complications.[96] NEWT detects newborns experiencing early rapid weight loss and alerts health professionals to evaluate adequacy of feeding before feeding complications occur.

Weight Loss Percentiles in Exclusively Breastfed, Vaginally Delivered (A) and Cesarean-Delivered (B) Newborns

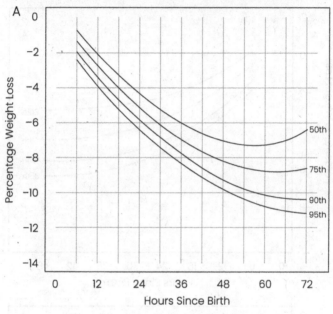

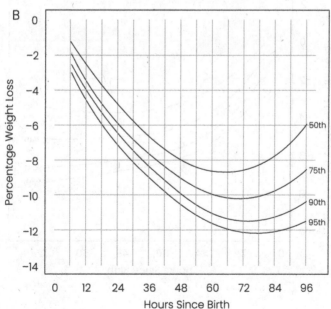

Weight Loss Percentiles in Exclusively Formula-Fed, Vaginally Delivered (A) and Cesarean-Delivered (B) Newborns

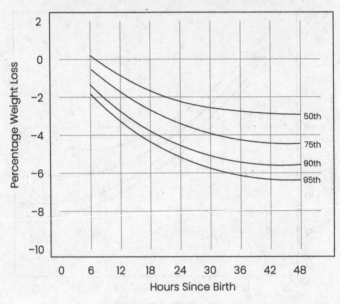

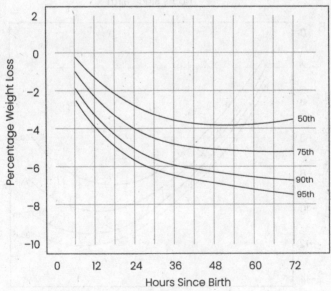

Since the NEWT data shows that exclusively breastfed newborns who lose weight the fastest (≥95th percentile) can lose 7 percent within twenty-four hours (a degree of weight loss that increases the risk of hyperbilirubinemia and hypernatremia), weighing exclusively breastfed newborns every twelve hours (instead of every twenty-four hours, as most hospitals do) may help identify those infants at risk for feeding complications earlier. Infants who have lost more weight than the 75th percentile according to the NEWT, or greater than 7 percent weight loss—particularly if there are signs of persistent hunger—should have a full clinical assessment of breastfeeding efficacy and breast milk supply, weighted feeds (to determine how much baby is getting from breastfeeding), and blood testing for hypoglycemia, hypernatremia, and hyperbilirubinemia.

One important caveat regarding using the NEWT as a trigger for finding feeding problems: While 75th percentile or greater weight loss indicates the need to assess adequacy of feeding, **average (or 50th percentile) weight loss on the NEWT (7–8 percent) is not sufficient to rule out whether an infant needs additional milk**. Remember, cases of hypernatremia and hyperbilirubinemia increase around 7–8 percent. Infants in the NEWT study were not universally screened for hypernatremia and few had glucose screening, so we don't actually know if the average weight loss was normal or safe. Since data now shows that hypernatremia, hyperbilirubinemia, and hypoglycemia are common even in exclusively breastfed newborns with average-appearing weight loss, the study's protocol likely missed these important feeding complications.[97] In fact, in a follow-up study of the same newborns, 4.3 percent of vaginally delivered and 2.1 percent of cesarean-delivered exclusively breastfed newborns were readmitted to the hospital, most for feeding problems like jaundice and dehydration, roughly double the rates found in the formula-fed group.[98]

This result means it is still possible for newborns to develop a feeding complication while having average weight loss per the NEWT. In fact, in a study of eleven previously healthy term breastfed newborns who developed severe hypoglycemia (≤20 mg/dL) due to poor milk intake between days 2 and 5, the infants lost anywhere from 0 to 16 percent of their birth weight, and five out of eleven lost less than 7 percent.[99] One possible reason: different newborns, as we've discussed, are born with different caloric reserves. A newborn with little reserve may not be able lose much weight without becoming starved and hypoglycemic. **Therefore, it is not enough to evaluate a newborn's weight loss percentile on the NEWT.** Signs of satisfaction and other markers of adequate feeding must be assessed before ruling out the need for further assistance and/or supplementation.

THE GLOBAL RISE IN HOSPITAL ADMISSIONS FOR COMPLICATIONS OF INSUFFICIENT FEEDING

We have spent the last few sections looking at how gaps in patient education and clinical guidelines, combined with a hyperfocus on exclusive breast-feeding, can lead to infant-feeding complications. These individual cases ultimately contribute to a larger epidemic of newborn hospitalizations. Multiple studies have shown an increase in admissions for newborn jaundice—the most common reason for newborn admission—as well as other feeding complications following the establishment of the Baby-Friendly Hospital Initiative in countries worldwide.[100] Whereas in 1986, before the BFHI, hyperbilirubinemia affected only 6.1 percent of healthy term newborns in the US,[101] it now affects approximately 30 percent.[102] Exclusive breastfeeding has been shown to be an independent risk factor for hypoglycemia admission,[103] and a rise in these admissions has been linked to BFHI hospital certification.[104] Increased admissions for hypernatremic dehydration have also been linked to implementation of an exclusive-breastfeeding hospital policy.[105] And since exclusive breastfeeding before milk comes in became standard practice, an entire system of follow-up visits, weight checks, and laboratory monitoring has become necessary to protect infants from the devastating consequences of insufficient feeding, complications that commonsense supplementation of breastfeeding previously prevented.[106]

This is particularly unfortunate in low- and middle-income countries (LMICs).[107] Exclusive breastfeeding with avoidance of supplemental feedings unless clearly medically necessary has also been heavily promoted in

LMICs despite long local traditions of prelacteal feeding before full milk production. In combination with minimal public awareness of newborn jaundice, many infants, especially those in families who cannot afford in-hospital deliveries, often receive little to no monitoring for jaundice and weight loss, leaving the most severely affected infants coming to the hospital at very late stages of acute bilirubin encephalopathy, resulting in high rates of severe disability and death.[108] Jaundice has been widely recognized as the leading cause of newborn hospital admissions in the first week of life and a major contributor to the prevalence of intellectual impairments, cerebral palsy, and other developmental disabilities across the globe.[109] Some of the worst cases of jaundice resulting in kernicterus occur in LMICs.[110] Even when excessive jaundice is identified, many hospitals have too few phototherapy machines to properly treat these infants, sometimes putting multiple babies under one lamp, each receiving suboptimal treatment.[111]

Internationally renowned jaundice expert Dr. Vinod Bhutani and colleagues estimated that in 2010, about 18 percent (24 million or almost 1 in 5) of the 134 million liveborn babies across the globe developed phototherapy-requiring jaundice and 481,000 late preterm and term newborns developed extreme hyperbilirubinemia (>25 mg/dL), resulting in 114,000 deaths and more than 63,000 survivors with moderate or severe irreversible brain injuries.[112] Those numbers may be overwhelming to contemplate, but every single one represents a family who will struggle with their newborn's entirely preventable disability for the rest of their lives. Bhutani and colleagues noted the significant contribution of suboptimal breastfeeding and dehydration to the global incidence of hyperbilirubinemia.

THE HAZARDS OF AGGRESSIVE EXCLUSIVE BREASTFEEDING PROMOTION AND INCOMPLETE PARENT EDUCATION

So far, the focus in addressing feeding complications has been to increase breastfeeding support. However, breastfeeding support alone cannot prevent all feeding complications, as it cannot eliminate the biological limitation of low milk supply. Furthermore, if the type of breastfeeding support a mother receives is biased toward avoiding supplementation, then a mother could be influenced to overlook the signs of insufficient feeding and to view even medically necessary supplementation as a threat to her breastfeeding efforts and her child's health.

Mistakes in health policy have been made throughout history, but a health policy focused on avoiding supplementation during a period when birthing mothers have the lowest milk supply available to fully feed their infants may be one of the most dangerous and farthest reaching. While these consequences may have been unintended, they still have a very real and, at times, devastating impact on families. We need a better systemic safety net, one that protects all infants from feeding complications—especially if families aren't fully informed. Even next-day office visits cannot prevent them if the complications occur at home.

Most parents today are provided little to no guidance upon discharge on how to recognize danger signs of underfeeding and when supplementing their breastfed infants is appropriate. Given the high rates of delayed lactogenesis II, this policy gap leaves more than one in five discharged exclusively breastfed newborns and almost *half* of first-born exclusively breastfed newborns at risk of feeding complications. This failure of the standard of care leaves exclusively breastfed newborns who run out of caloric and fluid reserves before their mother's milk comes in at risk for preventable brain injury and permanent disabilities. At *best*, it forces many infants to tolerate days of unnecessary hunger and thirst. This violates the ethical requirement to provide informed consent to patients and is a hideous oversight in how we are caring for new babies. It is unacceptable for medical organizations to put their desire to promote exclusive breastfeeding above their ethical obligation to ensure newborns are safe and free from hunger and thirst— especially when safe and successful breastfeeding *is* possible through temporary, judicious supplementation when babies show they need it.

FED IS BEST SAFE NEWBORN FEEDING GUIDELINES

Ensuring safe feeding for all infants requires objective criteria based on the best scientific data on long-term brain-development outcomes. It also requires parents, health professionals, and hospitals to monitor infants' behavior, weight, clinical signs, and blood work (if needed) using the most conservative thresholds to determine when supplementation is necessary to protect infant health. To read and download our guidelines for safe newborn feeding, scan the QR code.

PART 2
The Fed Is Best Guide to Safe and Optimal Infant Feeding

5

Before Birth: Preparing to Feed Your Baby

Now that we have covered the science that defines safe infant feeding and uncovered the reality beneath the myths around breastfeeding and formula feeding, we apply that knowledge to help you prepare for the birth of your baby. Ensuring the best feeding experience requires you to prepare during the months before delivery by learning basic infant-feeding skills, knowing how to recognize feeding problems, and coming up with a plan of how to manage them if they arise. Having health professionals and a health facility that support you and your informed choices are important as well.

The following is a guide on how to find the right health professionals, hospitals or birth facilities, and educational resources; how to document your infant-feeding goals and share them with your health professionals;

and what things you need to learn before you deliver. Keep in mind that not much in parenting goes exactly as planned. Flexibility is essential.

Use the QR code to access a helpful checklist of things to do or learn before birth, summarizing the topics in this chapter.

CHOOSE YOUR FEEDING PLAN

Most parents who pick up this book will already have some idea how they might want to feed their baby. Many choose a feeding plan based on what they are told about the health advantages and disadvantages of different feeding methods, their occupation, family life, previous experiences, and many other factors (read the beginnings of chapters seven through ten for some of the reasons people might choose different methods). Some take a wait-and-see approach; others are certain of their goals.

Here are the basic approaches:

Exclusive breastfeeding (EBF): your baby only gets milk directly from the breast from birth to six months; any medically necessary supplementation is done only with expressed or banked human milk (BHM).[1] Babies who have an effective nursing pattern and access to a full milk supply thrive with EBF.

Predominant breastfeeding (BF): supplementing with formula as needed, often for temporary episodes of low milk supply, with the aim of mostly breastfeeding long term.

Breastfeeding directly and feeding expressed breast milk (EBM) by bottle: also a form of EBF, commonly done by working mothers.

Combination breastfeeding and formula feeding (combo feeding or CF): direct nursing and feeding with EBM and/

or formula by bottle or supplemental nursing system (SNS; see page 141); common for those with a partial milk supply.

Exclusive Formula Feeding (EFF): baby is entirely fed formula by bottle.

Exclusively pumping and feeding EBM by bottle (EP): also a form of EBF commonly done when baby is unable to latch or if the lactating parent is averse to directly nursing.

Breastfeeding with predominant formula feeding at the breast: called "comfort nursing" or "dry nursing" for those with very limited or no milk supply who wish to nurse directly. This is done by feeding the available breast milk, then feeding formula at the breast with an SNS. This can be done to help bring a milk supply for nonlactating parents.

WHEN BREASTFEEDING IS NOT ADVISABLE

Though you may want to breastfeed, a few situations make breast-feeding inadvisable, like certain maternal infections or taking medication that is unsafe for a baby, or if the baby has certain medical conditions like galactosemia. Scan the QR code for a full list and consult with your doctor.

FIND YOUR INFANT-FEEDING SUPPORT TEAM

It's important to have a team that supports your infant-feeding goals well before delivery. This team can include your partner, family members, obstetrician or certified nurse midwife, pediatrician, family doctor, and/or lactation consultant (IBCLC) or certified lactation counselor (CLC).[2] Studies show that a partner's support plays a positive role in a mother's ability to sustain breastfeeding in particular.[3] Peer support groups can also be helpful, especially alongside professional support.[4]

High-quality support is nonjudgmental, inclusive, and attentive to the mental, emotional, and physical health of parents and baby alike.[5] Professionals absolutely must have a strong commitment to science and only recommend interventions that are supported by high-quality evidence, thus taking accountability for their recommendations.[6] Last, they should genuinely respect your informed choice to feed your baby in the way that works best for your family.

Obstetrician or Certified Nurse Midwife

Parents typically choose and visit their obstetrician or certified nurse midwife in the first trimester. Your obstetric provider should be knowledgeable about all feeding options. For parents who want to breastfeed, the provider should review any medical or psychosocial conditions that can affect breastfeeding and assess breast anatomy and growth. They should have a basic understanding of breastfeeding management and offer clear and conservative guidelines for preventing feeding complications. The provider should respectfully support your plan without pressure. Be wary of clinics or health providers that don't discuss insufficient feeding problems or who treat insufficient milk supply as either not real or so rare that it's not worthy of attention. Also, avoid providers that are willing to prescribe risky medications to increase milk supply (see chapter six).

Pediatricians and Family Practitioners

Many expectant parents also meet with prospective pediatricians or family practitioners before their baby's birth to decide who will become their baby's doctor. You may want to ask them these questions:

1. Do you provide inclusive and unbiased support for exclusive breastfeeding, combo feeding, and exclusive formula feeding families?

2. Is there a lactation consultant on staff who can assist me with breastfeeding and feeding problems under your guidance?

3. How do you evaluate, prevent, and treat insufficient feeding complications?

4. Do you use the Newborn Weight Tool (NEWT)?

5. What are your supplementing guidelines to prevent feeding complications? Are they the same as the hospital's guidelines?

6. Do you provide clinic visits the next day after discharge and/or weekend hours?

7. Do you have an after-hours line for urgent questions?

Lactation Professionals

If you plan to breastfeed, we recommend looking for a lactation consultant (LC)—either an International Board Certified Lactation Consultant (IBCLC) or a certified lactation counselor (CLC)—in the third trimester. IBCLCs typically have more education and experience than CLCs. Your LC should assess your medical history and learn your goals. They should help you identify your risk factors for breastfeeding challenges as early as possible and develop a clear and proactive plan with you to address them. Having a backup plan will give you the confidence you need to protect your milk supply *and* your baby if supplementation is needed, until breastfeeding problems can be addressed. Seek an LC with extensive experience helping mothers breastfeed successfully and safely through their challenges.

Ten Questions to Ask a Prospective LC

1. Can you describe your approach to helping families breastfeed?

2. How do you determine whether a newborn is getting enough milk, losing too much weight, or not gaining well?

3. Do you have a scale for doing pre- and postfeed weights?

4. What do you usually recommend if you see a baby who isn't getting enough milk?

5. If breastfeeding hurts, what do you usually recommend? What if those things don't work?

6. If it continues to hurt even if we have a "good latch" according to multiple LCs, how can you help me with my long-term breast-feeding goals?

7. What is your experience with bottles, pumping, and combo feed-ing? [Note: Even if you plan to exclusively breastfeed, asking this question can shed light on how flexible and patient-centered a lac-tation provider is.]

8. I'm concerned about getting enough sleep with a newborn. What do you usually recommend if I'm finding I need more sleep?

9. What are your recommendations about pacifiers for breastfed babies?

10. What are your recommendations about other baby/breastfeeding tools, such as pillows, lactation cookies, bedsharing, etc.?

Note that these are all open-ended questions. The purpose of asking these sorts of questions is to determine whether you and a professional will work well together. New parenthood can be one of the most vulnerable times in your life; it is essential to surround yourself with people who bring you comfort and confidence. It is important for your LC to help you breast-feed, but their primary concern should be the overall health and happiness of you and your child.

FIND TRUSTED SOURCES OF INFORMATION

You may notice as you ask questions about infant feeding that different peo-ple provide different answers, which can be frustrating. Infant feeding can be an emotionally charged topic, often colored by a professional's clinical and personal experiences, and many people have belief systems that influ-ence their answers.[7] You will have to decide what of this information rings true for you and what will work best for you and your family.

Formula- and Bottle-Feeding Information

There are few noncommercial resources with accurate and comprehensive information about formula and bottles. Sources on social media can be inaccurate; products are often marketed using statements not backed up by science. The CDC's (cdc.gov) and AAP's (healthychildren.org) sites are good but don't address all the questions parents have. Pediatricians are a great resource but they may not have unlimited time or be immediately available.

One source that provides independent formula information is the US-based formulasense.com, which was created by a pediatric registered dietitian and does not accept compensation of any kind from formula manufacturers. We have also done our best in chapters nine and eleven to present current evidence about formula and bottles.

Breastfeeding and Parenting Classes, Books, Websites, and Social Media Sites

Most hospitals offer free breastfeeding classes to new parents. While they provide valuable information about positioning, latching, and some newborn hunger cues, they should not be your only source of education. Some of the information presented may be incorrect (e.g., the small-stomach myth) or incomplete (e.g., no discussion of delayed or low milk production). Breastfeeding is rarely straightforward, and many mothers have told us their classes did not prepare them to recognize or solve common problems. Ultimately, breastfeeding classes provide a good introduction, but make sure to learn all the skills discussed in this book and our online resources.

The vast number of written resources on breastfeeding makes it difficult to recognize which use current science and which are false or downright dangerous. Breastfeeding books, classes, websites, and social media sites should be viewed *critically*—they often contain information based on ideology rather than science. Does the resource cite peer-reviewed articles to back their claims? Are the recommended interventions supported by randomized clinical trials (the best research method to show if something works)? Does it rely heavily on natural fallacy (e.g., glorifying "the biological norm") or treat common problems like low milk supply as rare or insignificant? Does the resource vilify formula or treat those who use it condescendingly? Some social media groups are full of shaming and judgment, and most do not have licensed health professionals to ensure that only safe advice is being given.

Breastfeeding resources should do the following:

- Be truthful, respectful, and inclusive of the spectrum of biological, psychological, and social circumstances that determine "best" infant feeding.
- Provide realistic expectations and ways to deal with feeding problems *before* they happen or become serious.
- Present recommendations backed by high-quality research (e.g., randomized controlled trials, systematic reviews), not just expert opinion or observational studies. Be wary of pseudoscience and thinly disguised opinion papers dressed up in the trappings of science. Being published in a peer-reviewed journal does not necessarily mean a study is high quality or that its conclusion is well supported by the data presented. Authors and peer reviewers, like anyone, have their own biases.

Be wary of resources that do the following:

- Minimize or ignore the risks of jaundice, dehydration, low blood sugar, excessive weight loss, or slow growth from poor feeding, or fail to give criteria for what is unsafe.
- Fail to provide a baby's daily caloric, fluid, or milk requirements.
- Broadly paint formula as substandard or a threat to breastfeeding without discussing the risks of feeding complications or the importance of supplementation when breast milk is not enough.

- Minimize parents' concerns about insufficient feeding, quickly label these concerns as "perceived" or imagined, or give false reassurance without offering objective criteria for adequate feeding.
- Discourage measuring objective data like weighted feeds, weight monitoring with growth charts, or pumping to estimate supply.

Unfortunately, the reason why the Fed Is Best Foundation exists and why over a million people support its mission is the complete absence of parent resources that provide adequate information on preventing infant-feeding complications. This is why hospitalizations for these conditions have increased and become routine. No parent would knowingly starve their child; it is through *disinformation and the omission of facts* in many current resources that this has become so common.

Remember that no resource is without bias, including ours. The bias of many breastfeeding resources is to promote EBF for every baby as the "biological norm." Our bias is to ensure safe and optimal outcomes for every child and family by recommending supplementation *before* medical complications occur, for babies who are hungry despite adequate time breastfeeding. Since the biological norm is that milk supply varies from insufficient to overabundant, we validate and support *every* clinically safe feeding method. With that, we recommend you read all the relevant chapters in this book and print out important tables before you deliver, and have a feeding plan written down to share with your delivery team.

LEARN ABOUT YOUR HOSPITAL OR BIRTH FACILITY'S POLICIES, LACTATION SERVICES, AND NURSERY CARE

Your hospital's maternity and lactation services and policies can significantly affect your family's feeding experience and outcome. Most hospitals follow the WHO's Ten Steps to Successful Breastfeeding. We will discuss in chapter seven the WHO's own assessment of how helpful (or not) the individual steps are for promoting breastfeeding. Keep this in mind as your hospital outlines their breastfeeding policies. Don't be shy about letting them know your preferences and asking if they will be supported. If you have options, choose the hospital or birthing facility that has the best services, most supportive and respectful staff and hospital policies, and lowest rates of newborn feeding-complication admissions. Here are a few questions to ask while you are touring the facility.

Questions to Ask If You Are Breastfeeding

Will I have access to a lactation consultant or infant-feeding specialist during my stay? When are they available?
A trained health professional should be available 24/7 to help mom and baby latch correctly within an hour after birth if mom and baby are healthy. Parents can't fully prepare for optimal latching with videos and books. Many hospitals have IBCLCs during regular business hours; some offer evening and weekend services. Mother–baby nurses are also trained to help get breastfeeding off to a good start and can often solve common problems after hours. Upon request, these health providers should be able to guide formula-feeding and combo-feeding families as well. You should have high-quality support that supports your infant-feeding goals while ensuring your baby gets enough to eat.

What if my baby is crying or nursing for hours and is not satisfied with breastfeeding? How will you determine if they are getting enough milk? What are your criteria for supplementation?
Many parents who have written to us have had their concerns about their infant's prolonged crying and nursing dismissed by health professionals as "normal," "cluster feeding," or "second night syndrome," only to find at the next weight check that they were right about their baby's hunger. Asking what the hospital protocol for assessing feeding problems is, and their criteria for supplementation, can help you decide if the hospital's policies can adequately protect your baby from feeding complications. Some detailed follow-up questions include: Do they supplement before a baby needs phototherapy? Do they supplement to satisfaction or do they restrict

supplemental volumes? Do they use the Pediatric Endocrine Society's glucose thresholds of 50 and 60 mg/dL or do they permit lower numbers before they consider supplementation medically necessary?

How are parent requests for formula handled when babies are hungry but do not meet supplementation criteria?

Hospitals have policies regarding formula requests for persistent hunger without medical complications. Some require counseling and a signed informed consent form (see two questions down). **Persistent signs of hunger despite frequent breastfeeding (after the first twenty-four hours)—even without meeting medical criteria—are enough to justify supplementation, according to the lead author of the Academy of Breastfeeding Medicine supplementation guidelines.**[8] (And note that the twenty-four-hour condition is based on her opinion, not evidence.) If supplementation is discouraged, yet you wish to do so, let hospital staff know that you are exercising your right as a parent to feed your baby as you choose.

Can healthy term breastfed babies who need supplementation get banked human milk?

Families concerned about the potential need for supplementation may prefer to supplement with BHM, which is an excellent option. Human milk banks screen breast milk donors for infectious diseases, medication, and drug use, among other risk factors, and donor milk is pasteurized to eliminate any remaining viruses and bacteria.

If you wish to supplement with BHM should the need arise, you may want to ask if it will be available to your baby, as some hospitals limit it to medically vulnerable infants.[9] If it is not available, rest assured that there have been no documented measurable differences in health outcomes between healthy term infants who are temporarily supplemented with formula versus those given human milk, nor is there any permanent or clinically significant difference in the gut microbiome (sometimes cited to discourage giving babies even a few teaspoons of formula).[10]

BEWARE OF INFORMALLY SHARED DONOR MILK

Donor milk obtained through informal sharing is not recommended by the AAP, CDC, or FDA, given the risk of infectious disease to your infant.[11] One study of 1,091 mothers interested in donating showed that about 3 percent were unknowingly positive for syphilis, hepatitis B or C, HTLV, or HIV.[12]

Does the hospital require a doctor's order or signed consent form to receive formula?
Hospital policies that require a physician's order for formula have caused families to experience unwanted delays in receiving the milk their baby needs. Some have had to wait for hours or have received only a fraction of their infant's need; others have been denied. Still others have been given formula by one staff member only to have it taken out of their room by another. Consequently, some infants have required NICU admission because of delayed or inadequate supplementation.

If you want to supplement your persistently hungry baby until your milk comes in, or if you want to combo-feed or exclusively formula-feed from the start, consider discussing this with your pediatrician and request an order or prescription for formula ahead of time, or bring your own. (Note: This is only to make it easier and more expedient for staff—you *always* have the right to feed your baby as you wish, and your baby has the right to sufficient food.)

You may be asked to sign an infant formula consent form. These are written solely to discourage supplementation with formula.[13] Many such forms state that giving *any formula,* even a small amount to relieve hunger, is linked to multiple long-term health problems, including allergies, diabetes, colitis, lower IQ, leukemia, and SIDS.[14] These exaggerated claims are based on observational studies—which, remember, do not prove causation—of babies whose mothers report feeding methods several months into infancy, *not* on babies who are temporarily supplemented (see chapter three). These forms provide no discussion of the greater risks of *failing* to supplement when breastfeeding is insufficient. Such consent forms have frightened parents into believing that even medically necessary supplementation is more dangerous than the feeding complications their infant may have developed. You have the right to decline signing these forms, and even if you decline, you should still expect your request for formula to be honored.

Is the hospital trying to increase their rates of exclusive breastfeeding before discharge?

Hospitals that have implemented the BFHI goal to increase EBF rates before discharge (meaning no formula to breastfed infants unless "medically necessary")* have had increased admissions for jaundice, hypoglycemia, and dehydration.[15] Since delayed and low milk production are common (affecting about 1 in 7 parents, according to former ABM president Dr. Alison Stuebe), so is the need for supplementation.[16] Parents are often discharged without education on appropriate supplementation and are thus unaware their babies aren't eating enough until complications occur. EBF at discharge has been associated with a two- to elevenfold increased risk of readmission compared to non-EBF newborns.[17] In contrast, five randomized clinical trials have shown that 10 mL (2 teaspoons) of supplementation of breastfed newborns with weight loss of 5 percent or more or greater than 75th percentile on the NEWT after every nursing session did not reduce breastfeeding rates at three months (and in one small study, supplementation actually improved them).[18] One of these studies found no differences at six months. Another found no supplemented newborn required hospital readmission. No trials have found that judicious supplementation reduces breastfeeding rates. While well intentioned, policies that focus on increasing EBF rates before discharge put undue pressure on health professionals and parents to avoid supplementation even when infants show obvious signs of persistent hunger.[19]

---

* The Joint Commission accredits hospitals, allowing them to receive reimbursement from Medicaid and Medicare.

Questions to Ask If You Are Planning to Formula-Feed Your Baby

Will I have to sign an informed consent form to get formula?
See discussion on page 122.

What kind of formula is used at your hospital?

Can I bring my own formula instead of using the hospital's?
If you want to use a different formula, you may also want to ask if there will be issues from hospital staff, who may be unaware that parents have that right. We strongly recommend using sterile nipples and ready-to-feed nursettes (2-ounce bottles made to be discarded after a single feed), which are sterile and already mixed. That will reassure your care providers that there will be no errors in preparation or contamination on their watch.

Questions to Ask If You Plan to Exclusively Pump

A few mothers know they want to only feed pumped milk in a bottle. Since this is less common, it's important to ask about it ahead of time. Not all hospitals have protocols for exclusive pumping. There may be gaps in the staff's knowledge base for answering pumping questions and troubleshooting.

Will a pump be available to me in the hospital from my first feeding or should I bring my own?

What facilities are available for cleaning and sanitizing pump parts?

Are trained staff available to help me pump exclusively?

Questions for All Families

Will I be able to access newborn nursery services if I am impaired due to pain, medication, or fatigue; am alone; or want to for any other reason?
Many families want to room in with their newborns, which we support. This can help parents learn their babies' hunger cues, and ensure adequate time feeding and bonding. However, due to the influence of the BFHI, families are being pressured to room in 24/7; families who have requested nursery care, especially those who are breastfeeding, are often counseled against doing so with the claim that it can impair breastfeeding.[20] The reality is that extreme exhaustion from labor and delivery is common. Some mothers are recovering from surgical births, taking pain medication, are extremely sleep deprived, and often without their partner overnight. Pressuring mothers to care for their newborns while exhausted or impaired has resulted in accidental falls and suffocation deaths of newborns.[21] It is also inhumane. Some who have asked for their baby to be sent to the nursery for just a few hours have been shamed or flat-out denied.[22] Many hospitals have closed their nurseries, ostensibly to encourage breastfeeding.[23]

Newborn nurseries are a safety net for babies and parents. Not every birthing mother will have a support person with her around the clock. If you feel unable to safely care for your newborn due to exhaustion, nursery services should be available to facilitate your recovery and protect your baby. While you may be counseled against using nursery services, hospital staff must provide it to you if you still want it.[24] Babies can be brought back to feed and resume rooming in when you are rested. If you are refused nursery care, ask to speak with the charge nurse, and insist they document their denial of your request after you stated that you are at risk of falling asleep while caring for your newborn alone.

Rooming in 24/7 has been shown to have no significant effect on sustained breastfeeding rates at three to six months, according to the 2017 WHO breastfeeding guidelines.[25] Therefore, pressuring parents to room in 24/7 puts them at risk of dropping or falling asleep with their babies for *no proven benefit*. It should never be interpreted as a strict mandate. Although

BFHI advocates would insist it is a recommendation and not a mandate, in practice it is being interpreted that way.[26] Recovering parents deserve rest, and only they know when they are able to safely care for their babies alone.

> I think with the loss of nurseries, both non-BFHI and BFHI hospitals have placed newborn care onto parents from the moment the baby is delivered. Babies are born, then to belly for skin-to-skin. Skin-to-skin happens in the operating room while they are still closing up the incision on the mother, then skin-to-skin for the two-hour recovery time. Then they go straight to the room, where mothers are expected to care for their infant. No one gets a pass with baby care, even if a mother had a three-day induction, pregnancy-induced hypertension and is on magnesium, six hours of pushing, a crash c-section, a third-degree tear, 1000 ml blood loss, or postpartum hemorrhage. It. Does. Not. Matter.
>
> —Elaine, neonatal nurse practitioner at a Baby-Friendly Hospital

What percentage of healthy term newborns in your hospital require phototherapy or get admitted for jaundice, dehydration, hypernatremia, or hypoglycemia?

Hospitals should be tracking rates of moderate jaundice and phototherapy admissions, which include those that occur during the birth hospitalization and after discharge, according to the Joint Commission's Perinatal Care Measure PC–06. Some hospitals don't receive readmissions and refer patients to other hospitals, resulting in incomplete data. Since about 75 percent of excessive jaundice and phototherapy occur before discharge, this is still useful information.[27] If they do not know, you can ask the nurse manager of the birth unit for an estimate of how many healthy term newborns are admitted for jaundice, hypoglycemia, or dehydration per week on average. This number will give you an idea of how effective the hospital's policies are in preventing feeding complications; the closer it is to zero, the better.

Newborn comfort and safety, and the prevention of medical complications, should be the primary goals of any hospital and health professional. Staff should respect your feeding goals and give you evidence-based advice to keep your baby safely fed. If you are exclusively breastfeeding, you should expect honesty and objective evidence when you ask if your baby is getting enough nutrition. In the absence of blood tests, the best ways to know if your baby is being adequately fed in the first few days are your baby's hunger and fullness cues and their weight loss pattern on the NEWT tool. Infant swallows and diaper counts (especially in the first four days) are *only clues*—not accurate measures of feeding.[28] If you wish to supplement your persistently hungry baby with formula or wish to combo-feed until your milk is in, you are making choices that have a rational and scientific basis, and they should be respected and provided without your being lectured about the alleged risks. Failing to provide adequate nutrition carries far greater risks than the purported risks of formula commonly listed in hospital informed consent forms, and you have the right to protect your infant from these conditions.

LEARN THE SIGNS OF A WELL-FED NEWBORN

It is important to learn the signs of adequate versus inadequate feeding, which are extensively covered in chapters four and six. We recommend downloading and printing the tables and checklists (use the QR code on page 149), as well as the Fed Is Best Feeding Plan, accessible at the QR code here, which also provides a helpful hospital log to track your feeding sessions, weight, and bilirubin and glucose levels.

LEARN HOW TO CALCULATE WEIGHT LOSS PERCENTAGE AND USE THE NEWBORN WEIGHT TOOL

As discussed in chapter four, weight is tracked after birth and can be plotted on the Newborn Weight Tool (NEWT), which compares your newborn's weight to other healthy term newborns within the first seventy-two hours. This helps identify newborns with possible feeding problems, which can result in excessive weight loss, which is currently defined as greater than the 75th percentile on the graph. Your nurse or doctor should be able to tell you what percentage of their birth weight your baby has lost and show you their NEWT percentile. However, you can also create this graph yourself, by putting your baby's weights (and the times they were measured) into the NEWT at www.newbornweight.org; the site also offers a tutorial on its use. This tool is available for newborns who are breastfed or formula fed exclusively. If you are combo feeding and supplementing to satisfaction, use the formula-fed graph, as your baby will more likely follow that pattern.

Below are examples of reassuring and concerning NEWT graphs for a vaginally delivered breastfed newborn (see pages 101–102 for the NEWT graphs for EBF and EFF babies).

Reassuring NEWT graph

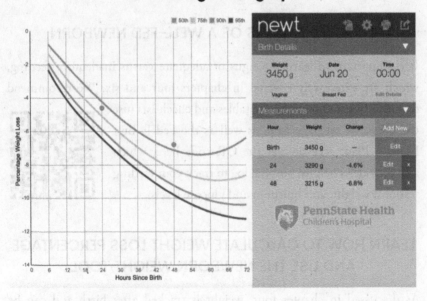

Concerning NEWT graph

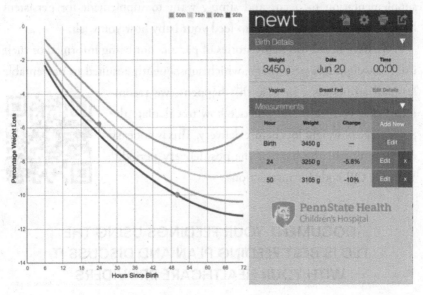

The topmost, 50th-percentile line indicates average weight loss; the second topmost, 75th-percentile line indicates that your baby has lost more weight than 75 percent of babies at that hour of age. According to the ABM, a percentile higher than the 75th is considered an indication for a feeding evaluation. Such weight loss can be a sign of a feeding problem that requires medically necessary supplementation.[29]

Remember, however, that the NEWT can only tell you how your baby compares to other babies at the same hour of life and mode of birth (vaginal or cesarean), and "normal" weight loss on the graph does not guarantee absence of a feeding complication. Those conditions can only be excluded based on your newborn's feeding behavior and laboratory data like glucose, bilirubin, and sodium levels. Note also that excessive jaundice and high sodium dehydration increase at 7 percent weight loss.[30] Therefore, we recommend supplementation at or above the 75th percentile weight loss, unless glucose, bilirubin, or sodium levels are confirmed to be normal and your baby appears satisfied. If those lab numbers are abnormal, regardless of weight loss percentage, supplementation should be given to satisfaction to correct them. And if you do not want to wait for medical indications for supplementation to occur and simply want to supplement for persistent hunger, it is always your right to feed your baby how you wish.

We have heard too many stories of parents not being informed of their infant's weight loss percentage, which subsequently resulted in preventable hospital admissions. In case this happens, we recommend that you learn and practice how to calculate the percentage of weight loss before delivery. This is not easy to figure out in the haze of the postdelivery period.[31] Scan the QR code for instructions.

DOCUMENT YOUR FEEDINGS USING THE FED IS BEST FEEDING PLAN AND DISCUSS IT WITH YOUR HEALTHCARE PROVIDERS

Having an infant-feeding plan can help you communicate your infant-feeding goals with your health providers before delivery. For breastfeeding parents, it communicates what you would like to do if the unexpected occurs and you and/or your infant require extra support with breastfeeding technique, positioning, supplementation, and/or nursery services. For combo-feeding or exclusive formula-feeding families, it can prevent unwanted lectures during this special time.

To help you, we have created a printable infant-feeding plan at the QR code below. Sharing this with your health team will make them aware that you are informed of the risks and benefits of different methods of infant feeding and what you would like to do in case feeding challenges occur. This is an important document that helps protect your and your baby's right to safe infant-feeding support and management, and we suggest you ask the hospital to put it in your baby's chart, just like your birth plan. It includes a crib sign that summarizes your infant-feeding plan for your health providers.

IF YOU PLAN TO BREASTFEED . . .

LEARN HOW TO POSITION AND LATCH YOUR BABY

Before you give birth, it is important to learn about different breastfeeding positions and how to help a newborn baby latch effectively onto your breast. The best breastfeeding position is the one that you find comfortable and that enables your baby to easily latch on and feed without causing nipple pain, which will vary with the baby's age and with the mother's and baby's anatomy.

There are countless resources, but we recommend going to our full guide on breastfeeding position and latch online at the QR code. We encourage you to review it while using a doll or teddy bear to help with visualization and muscle memory.

LEARN ABOUT AND PURCHASE A BREASTFEEDING PILLOW

A breastfeeding pillow can provide very helpful support while learning to position and latch. For the first few weeks, most parents like a firm, flat pillow that wraps around their torso to provide back support. Pillows that are rounded (like an inner tube) are often not ideal postpartum; the curved surface can be unstable for holding the baby's head and body, which can affect the latch and cause sore nipples.

LEARN HOW TO HAND-EXPRESS COLOSTRUM

Colostrum is typically thicker than mature milk and is sometimes more effectively expressed by hand than with a breast pump. Therefore, before you give birth (but no earlier than 37 weeks and only with your obstetric provider's approval, as it can trigger premature contractions),[32] it is important to learn how to hand-express your breasts for colostrum. You can even collect and freeze it to bring to the hospital for supplementation (although additional supplements will be needed if there is a medical issue like newborn hypoglycemia).[33]

We also recommend hand expression before each feed to check for the presence of ample colostrum. While it's a rarely talked-about phenomenon, some mothers produce little to no colostrum; others produce less on the second day.[34] Either of these can pose a health risk to exclusively breastfed newborns. When there is no observable colostrum, we cannot simply *assume* that a baby is transferring milk, because their health depends on the confirmed presence of colostrum.

There are other benefits to learning how to hand-express colostrum. In case of separation from your infant, you can collect colostrum for later feeding. Gentle hand massage during breastfeeding can also help a newborn who has weak or ineffective suck to obtain colostrum. And a similar technique can be used during pumping to increase the yield of breast milk from a session.

You can access our guide to hand-expressing by scanning the QR code.

BUY A BREAST PUMP AND LEARN HOW TO USE IT

Few mothers are taught how to use a breast pump before they deliver. Knowing how to pump before you enter the haze of the perinatal period will help you be more prepared if it is needed or desired.

One important reason to learn to pump ahead of time is that sometimes circumstances around delivery require mother and infant to be separated, and pumping can both protect your milk supply and allow your baby to still receive your milk. In those cases, hospital pumps will usually be available. However, some hospitals will only provide a pump if there is a medical indication recognized by the facility (e.g., need for intensive care). Therefore, consider bringing your own pump with you just in case. As just discussed, you can also hand-express colostrum, as an alternative.

IDENTIFY YOUR RISKS FOR BREASTFEEDING CHALLENGES AND DEVELOP AN ACTIONABLE FEEDING PLAN

CDC data from 2019 show 83 percent of US mothers initiate breastfeeding, yet only 56 percent are still breastfeeding at six months, and 36 percent at twelve months.[35] Multiple barriers often result in much shorter breastfeeding durations than intended, including:[36]

- inexperience with breastfeeding.
- poor family and social support.
- emotional barriers.
- psychosocial challenges like addiction, PTSD, sexual trauma, depression, and anxiety.
- employment barriers (lack of workplace accommodations, family leave, or affordable childcare).
- lack of access to quality health services and affordable breastfeeding support.
- maternal or infant medical conditions.
- lactation problems (milk supply, pain, breast anatomy, prior surgery, difficulty with latch).

It is important to take inventory of barriers you're already aware will apply to you, so you can plan how to address them. "Risk" only means there is an increased probability of a problem happening, not that one absolutely will. But, if a problem *does* happen, many women can still successfully breastfeed. Being prepared with a plan will help you do so.

The Most Common Breastfeeding Challenge: Delayed Lactogenesis II

Like all biological processes, the ability to produce breast milk varies across the population and over time. Breasts begin to change within weeks of conception, often becoming more tender. Over the course of pregnancy, breasts grow as mammary glands proliferate in preparation for milk production. Breasts that produce a full milk supply commonly grow symmetrically, more than one cup size, in a round, nontubular fashion without too wide a gap in between (your lactation professional should be able to assess this). Having smaller breasts does not mean you will have low supply, as many such moms can and do exclusively breastfeed. But atypical breast growth and appearance are signs of potential impaired lactation that your health professionals should monitor.

Colostrum is typically produced starting mid-pregnancy and available for feeding at birth. Progesterone, a hormone produced by the placenta during pregnancy, inhibits full milk production until the baby and placenta are delivered. Delivery of the full placenta is crucial to milk production, as those who retain even one fragment can fail to undergo lactogenesis II. After delivery, progesterone levels begin to plummet, and the hormones prolactin and oxytocin are released in response to an infant suckling at the breasts, the combination of which triggers milk production.

Ideally, the onset of full milk production, or when "milk comes in," occurs two to three days after delivery, and is typically experienced as a noticeable fullness of the breasts corresponding with higher milk-volume production. When functioning optimally for exclusive breastfeeding, your milk supply will match or slightly exceed your baby's demand and increase as your infant signals the need for more nutrition by removing more milk.

However, lactating parents produce different amounts of milk, have different storage capacities, and have varying biological limits. While parents are often taught that breastfeeding works near perfectly if you follow certain rules, the reality is that nothing about biology, including lactation, works perfectly at the rates we are led to believe.

One of the most common breastfeeding challenges, and the one most likely to put a newborn at risk of insufficient feeding, is delayed lactogenesis II.[37] It is critical to get ahead of this because what happens in the first week can impact the rest of your breastfeeding journey.

WHAT IS DELAYED LACTOGENESIS II AND WHO IS AFFECTED?

The term "lactogenesis II" refers to the onset of significantly increased milk production. A delay in this onset of greater than seventy-two hours after birth is referred to as delayed lactogenesis II, or DLII.[38] It can result in excessive newborn weight loss and other feeding complications that require medically necessary supplementation in exclusively breastfed newborns. DLII occurs in about 22 percent of healthy mothers delivering full term, 34–44 percent of first-time moms,[39] and around half in those with higher BMI[40] or unplanned cesareans.[41] It is unclear why DLII occurs, but research suggests it may be related to higher levels of maternal physical stress and exhaustion that can occur due to adverse circumstances during labor and delivery (e.g., prolonged labor).[42]

There are several risk factors for developing DLII, the most common of which we've listed below. In a 2010 study, researchers concluded that "the prevalence of [DLII] has reached epidemic proportions in the United States."[43]

List of Risk Factors for Delayed Lactogenesis II Before Delivery[44]

- First-time mother
- Advanced maternal age (≥30 years old)
- Diabetes
- Hypertension
- Pre-pregnancy BMI > 27
- Infertility
- History of low milk supply; delayed (>72 hours) or failed lactogenesis II
- Hormone problems: hypothyroidism, hypopituitarism
- Polycystic ovarian syndrome
- Prior breast surgery/injury/piercings
- Hypoplasia/insufficient glandular tissue (IGT)—minimal growth of breast tissue during pregnancy, tubular or asymmetric breasts

- Flat/inverted nipples
- Smoking
- Sickle cell disease
- Autoimmune diseases: multiple sclerosis, Crohn's, ulcerative colitis, lupus, rheumatoid arthritis

Percent of Mothers Who Develop
Delayed Lactogenesis II[45]

	% Who Develop DLII
All healthy mothers delivering a healthy term baby	22
First-time mothers	34–44
First-time mothers ≥ 30 years old	58.5
Mothers with flat or inverted nipples	44–56
Mothers with pre-pregnancy BMI ≥ 30	57.9

List of Risk Factors for Delayed Lactogenesis II Around Delivery[46]

- Cesarean section
- Complicated/prolonged labor > 12 hours
- Prolonged "pushing" stage of labor > 1 hour
- Maternal or infant medical complications
- Preterm baby (< 37 weeks gestation)
- Small-for-gestational-age baby
- Large-for-gestational-age baby
- Excessive blood loss (>500 mL) during delivery, need for transfusion
- Retained placenta

Percent of Mothers with Perinatal Risk Factors Who Develop Delayed Lactogenesis II[47]

Risk Factor for DLII	% Who Develop DLII
Stage II (pushing phase) labor lasting > 1 hour	36
Scheduled cesarean delivery	27
Urgent/emergent cesarean delivery	56
Birth weight ≥ 7 pounds, 15 ounces in first-time mothers	59
Maternal BMI 25.0–29.9 for first-time mothers (at day 7 postpartum)	44.8
Maternal BMI > 27 (at day 14 postpartum)	33
Maternal BMI > 30 for first-time mothers (at day 7 postpartum)	54

Some resources state milk coming in three to five days after delivery is "normal."[48] While this may be *common*, it is not safe for human babies to subsist on teaspoons of colostrum for three to five days. Remember also that the seventy-two-hour definition for delayed lactogenesis II is an *arbitrary* cutoff to help researchers study the phenomenon. It is possible for a newborn to develop feeding complications even if milk comes in before seventy-two hours, because mothers produce different amounts of colostrum and babies are born with different caloric and fluid reserves.

WAYS TO PREPARE IF YOU HAVE RISK FACTORS FOR DELAYED LACTOGENESIS II

Fortunately, DLII can be managed with optimization of breastfeeding technique and temporary supplementation until milk comes in; we'll discuss these in the next chapter. Here, we offer a few ways you can prepare to prevent feeding problems, in case you have any of the risk factors just discussed.

First-Time Mothers

As we've seen, up to 44 percent of healthy, first-time mothers experience DLII.[49] These mothers have the added challenge of being the least experienced at breastfeeding and recognizing infant hunger. The best ways to prepare as a first-time mother are to:

1. Watch videos on breastfeeding latch and positioning to familiarize yourself with the mechanics of breastfeeding.
2. Watch videos of hungry newborn babies and learn the signs of adequate versus inadequate feeding.
3. Learn about manual expression of colostrum and breast pumping in case breastfeeding is ineffective and colostrum needs to be fed by syringe.
4. Make an infant-feeding plan in case you develop DLII, so you can be confident that your baby is sufficiently fed even if it occurs (see the QR code on page 127).

Inverted and Flat Nipples

Inverted nipples are nipples that turn inward rather than pointing out, something that occurs in about 2–10 percent of women and can make effective latch difficult. Inverted nipples can range from slightly dimpled or flat, and correctable with suction, to deeply inverted and resistant to stretching. The more elastic the nipples are, the easier they are to correct.

Various tools and exercises have been promoted to treat inverted nipples prenatally; however, research has shown either that these are ineffective[50] or the data has been inadequate.[51] Some helpful strategies after birth include:

- Use a suction device for flat/inverted nipples, such as a Latch Assist or Supple Cups nipple extractor.
- Before feeding, pump your breasts for one to two minutes to temporarily stretch out the nipple and make it easier to grasp.

If neither of these approaches work, a nipple shield can be used to provide a teat for the baby to grasp. Nipple shields are made of thin silicone and come in different sizes and shapes; they should be measured for proper fit. Scan the QR code to learn more about nipple shields. Some mother–baby couplets are eventually able to latch and suck without the nipple shield. For others, a nipple shield is required for the full duration of breastfeeding. Whatever works for you and your baby is what you should continue doing. While there is a common perception that nipple shields can impair transfer of milk and threaten supply, a newer study has shown that they do not affect sucking strength or milk removal.[52]

If you have flat or inverted nipples, we suggest meeting with an LC prenatally to discuss strategies.

BODY MASS INDEX

High body mass index (BMI > 25) increases the risk for delayed DLII for various reasons. One may be the 1.3- to 3-fold higher rate of cesarean section among that group.[53] Alternatively, the increased risk may be related to hormonal factors like insulin resistance,[54] lower estrogen, higher androgen levels,[55] and lower prolactin response.[56] Those with larger breasts may also have difficulties with latching and positioning and thus have less effective milk removal. Helpful strategies include:

1. Striving for healthy weight gain during pregnancy.
2. Optimizing chronic medical conditions (e.g., diabetes) with your obstetric provider.
3. Working closely with your LC to ensure optimal latch and positioning.
4. Using breastfeeding positions such as the football hold, side-lying, or sitting with the weight of the breasts supported on a firm surface or with a small towel rolled beneath them to lift the nipples for improved latching.
5. If needed, using a mirror or phone camera to help you see your nipple and your baby's mouth while latching.

INSUFFICIENT GLANDULAR TISSUE

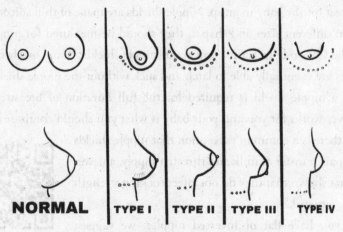

Insufficient glandular tissue

Breast hypoplasia, or insufficient glandular tissue (IGT), is a condition resulting in underdevelopment of breast glandular tissue. There are no studies that have determined the true prevalence of IGT, but it can cause low, scant, or absent breast milk despite efforts to increase supply.[57] Hypoplastic breasts are widely spaced, asymmetric, tuberous, or sac-like breasts, often with large areolas.[58] During pregnancy, IGT breasts do not increase in size as expected (see page 153).

All expectant mothers should be examined prenatally for potential IGT. Those with suspected IGT who still wish to breastfeed should closely follow the Fed Is Best Guidelines for Sufficient Breastfeeding in chapter six (page 153), as well as the following:

1. Have a supplementation plan before delivery until you know how much milk you will produce.
2. If you are producing little to no colostrum, consider supplementing breastfeeding earlier (after adequate time nursing to stimulate milk production).
3. If you want to supplement at the breast, we recommend trying a supplemental nursing system (SNS) to encourage direct

latching and increase the stimulus for milk production (see box below).

4.   See "Ways to Prepare If You Have Risk Factors for Delayed Lacto-genesis II" on page 137.

Note that once milk comes in and your baby has learned to nurse effectively, combination feeding will likely need to continue, whether through an SNS or bottle feeding. Some parents with IGT have been prescribed triple-feeding regimens (breastfeed, supplement, then pump) in an attempt to stimulate a full supply, but such a grueling regimen is ineffective for IGT, can give unrealistic expectations, and can ultimately compromise breastfeeding by making it unsustainable. For mothers with IGT, combination feeding (see chapter ten) can be a rewarding way to breastfeed.

WHAT IS A SUPPLEMENTAL NURSING SYSTEM?

An SNS is a device for mothers with IGT or low milk supply that uses a tube and a reservoir to supplement your baby at the breast. It ensures a well-fed baby while providing additional stimulation for milk pro-duction and encouraging the baby to continue latching. It can be homemade (which is more economical) or purchased, and may be used the first day if needed.

For those with risk factors for low milk supply, it's a good idea to become familiar with setting up an SNS before delivery; consider con-sulting an LC. An SNS should be cleaned and sterilized similar to bottles (see page 283). If an SNS system is not desirable, supplementing with a bottle is still a good option.

For more information on supplemental nurs-ing systems and how to use them, scan the QR code.

"

I didn't make enough breast milk for my first baby and was diagnosed with IGT. I used an SNS immediately with my subsequent
babies and was able to breastfeed them both for over a year . . .
Overall, it was a rewarding experience for me and my babies.

—Adrienne Rafuse

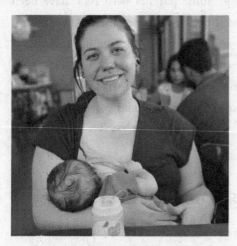

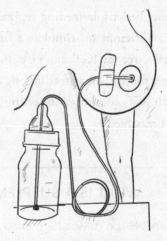

*Alleigh Cooper happily breastfeeds
her baby with a homemade
supplemental nursing system.*

*A homemade supplemental
nursing system*

DECIDE ON HOW YOU WANT TO SUPPLEMENT
SHOULD IT BECOME NECESSARY

It is important to consider ahead of time how you want to supplement your
infant should the need arise. The ABM recommends supplementing with
expressed breast milk (EBM) first, then banked human milk (BHM), then
formula as the last resort.[59] While we've seen how this bias against formula
is based on poor interpretation of the evidence, if you would *like* to supplement with BHM, this is an absolutely healthy option that is sometimes
available. Other parents are uncomfortable with supplementing with BHM
or prefer to reserve it for medically vulnerable infants. Supplementation

with your own expressed colostrum is also an option, but has been shown to be ineffective at correcting low blood sugar since it does not meet a baby's full caloric requirement.[60] Formula is also a healthy option for supplementation, and hospitals typically carry one brand of cow's milk formula. Other formula options are available, but you may have to bring your own if you want a different kind (see page 230 for options). Remember, however, that the type of milk you choose does not matter as much as how *much* you supplement with.

How Much Supplemental Milk Is Needed Per Feed?

There is much debate over the volume of supplemental milk that should be given for breastfed newborns who need it. Unfortunately, current recommendations can depend on the goal of the advising organization (e.g., increasing exclusive breastfeeding rates), rather than science. Prior to the BFHI, there were no rules for the amount that babies should be supplemented. Infants were generally fed to satisfaction; if they were breastfed, they were supplemented if they were hungry for more. Research on breastfed newborns supplemented to satisfaction (typically about 30–50 mL [1–1.7 fluid oz] per feeding for a 3 kg [6 lb, 10 oz] newborn) until milk came in found that rates of excessive jaundice *plummeted*, from previously reported rates of 30–35 percent to 1.3 percent.[61] Rates of jaundice requiring phototherapy fell from previously reported rates of 2.4–14 percent of newborns to only 0.3 percent. These infants had extremely low rates of weight loss exceeding 7 percent (0.4 percent of infants). Compare that to the currently reported 10–18 percent of exclusively breastfed newborns who lose greater than 10 percent.[62] This is a stunningly positive result, but parents are rarely told about this. **In plain words, newborns know when they are hungry and when they are full, and if fed to satisfaction, they will regulate their own bodies to prevent or correct complications of insufficient feeding.**

It may be helpful to know that the volume of the term newborn stomach has been scientifically measured at around 20 mL,[63] which makes a supplemental volume of 15 mL, repeated as needed, a reasonable starting point. No scientific data supports the safety of supplementing newborns who have a medical need with small volumes like 2–10 mL on day 1, 5–15 mL on day 2, and so forth, as recommended by the ABM, since it does not meet their full nutritional requirement.[64] Such small volumes will only perpetuate the underfeeding and dehydrating conditions that caused the feeding complication(s) to begin with.

How Do You Feed Supplemental Milk?

For years, the Ten Steps to Successful Breastfeeding recommended avoiding bottles for medically necessary supplementation. But as of the latest revision of the World Health Organization guidelines, after extensive review of the scientific literature, there was insufficient evidence to support this recommendation, leading the expert panel to drop the recommendation. Therefore, if you are breastfeeding and need to supplement, using a bottle with a slow-flow nipple should not impair breastfeeding (see page 274 for more on nipple types). A curved-tip oral syringe or a nipple without the bottle may be more useful for colostrum feeds less than 15 mL, since bottles cause waste from milk adhering to their walls. Spoons and cups are also options but can cause spills. A bottle may be useful for 15 to 30 mL feeds. For larger-volume supplementation (>30 mL), a bottle or an SNS is an option (see pages 141 and 262).

IF YOU PLAN TO COMBO-FEED
FROM THE FIRST FEED...

Parents who plan to combination-feed need to prepare in the same way as both breastfeeding and formula-feeding parents. Every chapter of this book will help you.

It's very important to discuss your plan with your obstetric provider and your health professionals where you deliver. You may receive counseling against combo feeding, but know that many families choose this to prevent hunger and feeding complications until breast milk satisfies their infants, which are valid reasons. Some birthing parents with risk factors for newborn hypoglycemia, like diabetes, choose this to reduce the risk of hypoglycemia.

So long as your baby is nursing well *at least* every three hours for around ten to fifteen minutes each breast, or you are manually expressing colostrum/pumping for the same if separated, you should adequately stimulate your breasts to produce milk. Remember to bring your own pump, as some facilities do not provide one unless it is medically indicated.

IF YOU PLAN TO FORMULA-FEED EXCLUSIVELY FROM THE FIRST FEED . . .

Research and decide what kind of formula you wish to use and whether you want to use the hospital's formula or an alternative. Know that it is okay to use one formula, then switch to another as long as it is the same type of formula (see page 230). Feed half an ounce (15 mL) at a time to satisfaction. Read more about expected volumes of feeds on page 243. It is also important to inform your health professionals of your plan to formula-feed ahead of delivery, as you may receive counseling against formula feeding. Just state your informed choice plainly, and they should honor it.

BREASTFEEDING AND PARENTING CLASSES ARE NOT ENOUGH

Parents often underestimate the amount of time and effort they need to prepare to feed their baby. Whether you will be breastfeeding or formula feeding, going to classes and relying on instruction at the time of delivery is frankly not enough to prepare you, especially if challenges arise.

We strongly believe that every birthing parent who wants to breastfeed can be supported in a way that maximizes their ability to succeed, regardless of how much milk they ultimately produce. If we can abandon rigid and incorrect assumptions about breastfeeding and change how we think about achieving the best outcomes for parents and their babies, then perhaps we can help families reach their breastfeeding goals in a healthy and sustainable manner. We believe combo-feeding and exclusive formula-feeding families also should be supported in their informed choice without unnecessary shaming or lecturing about the supposed dangers of formula feeding.

We further believe that parents are ideally positioned to determine what best infant feeding looks like for their baby, themselves, and their family, as long as they receive complete and unbiased information on all their feeding options and are taught to respond to challenges with realistic and judgment-free support. But to achieve this, we must prevent feeding complications for *every* infant. This requires parents and health professionals to recognize and take seriously the signs of feeding problems and take steps to diagnose them through objective means like weighing, blood testing, measuring milk supply and infant intake, and supplementing *before* unsafe conditions occur. This requires far more monitoring than is commonly offered in most hospitals—which we will discuss in the next chapter.

6

The First Few Days: How to Ensure Sufficient Feeding

The first days after birth are critical for establishing both breastfeeding and formula feeding. They are also when problems with insufficient feeding are most likely to occur. Therefore, knowing how to recognize adequate versus inadequate feeding are vital parenting skills—ones you should learn before arriving at your birth facility. Although this chapter is called "The First Few Days," you should not wait until then to read it.

Much of this chapter is geared toward parents who plan to feed exclusively at the breast, because their infants will need greater attention to ensure sufficient feeding, as they are prone to losing more weight than combo-fed and formula-fed newborns. However, all newborns need careful monitoring to ensure sufficient feeding, and the sections on adequate versus inadequate feeding, discharge planning, the first pediatric visit, and newborn milk requirements also apply to formula-fed, combo-fed, and expressed milk–fed babies.

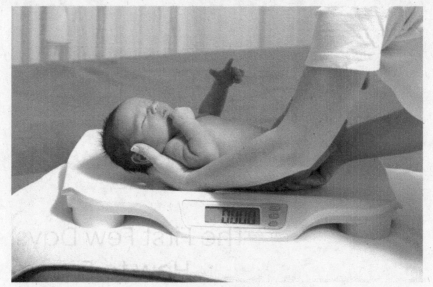

Monitoring infant weight is one important way to ensure adequate feeding.

In this chapter, we discuss how to evaluate your newborn's feeding after birth and provide information not included in most breastfeeding and parenting manuals. Until now, some of this has only been accessible to health professionals.

THE NORMAL FEEDING CYCLE

It's important to know what to expect from an adequately fed newborn as they feed throughout the day, so you can recognize when something is amiss. The typical pattern looks like this:

1. Baby shows signs of hunger by rooting, putting their hands in their mouth, fussing, and finally crying.
2. Baby nurses actively for about ten to fifteen minutes on each breast if breastfeeding, and fifteen to twenty minutes if formula-feeding. Once satisfied, they should release their latch from the nipple.
3. Baby shows hunger cues two to three hours later, indicating the need to feed again.

If a baby gets slightly less milk than what makes them full, they may want to feed a little earlier than three hours later. Feeding more frequently than every two hours and prolonged feedings (>30 minutes) throughout the day may be signs of a feeding problem that requires further evaluation.

MONITORING SIGNS OF ADEQUATE VERSUS INADEQUATE FEEDING

The first few days can be a sleep-deprived haze for parents, so logging your feedings can help you and your health professionals pick up on these early feeding problems. The hospital feeding log in the Fed Is Best Feeding Plan (see page 127 for a QR code to download this plan) can help you monitor your baby's feeding times and duration, their behavior, percentage weight loss, NEWT percentiles, blood test results, and other important data, which can help you and your health providers determine whether feeding is going well. (As discussed in chapter four, low blood glucose and high bilirubin can be signs of inadequate caloric intake. High blood sodium is caused by low body fluid from inadequate milk intake.) We also recommend printing the following tables, which are available at the QR code.

What Is Considered a Good Versus an Ineffective Breastfeeding Session?

Good Breastfeeding Session	Ineffective Breastfeeding Session
1. Baby is actively sucking and swallowing with a few short breaks, for at least 10–15 minutes on each breast. 2. Baby is satisfied after feeding.	1. Baby is latched but mostly sleeping while on the breast. 2. Baby does not sustain sucking or swallowing. 3. Baby must be frequently awakened to keep them latched or swallowing.

A Well-Fed Newborn . . .

- ❏ Is content after feedings.
- ❏ Is able to sleep for 2–3 hours between feedings.
- ❏ Wakes for feedings every 2–3 hours.
- ❏ Actively feeds during the entire feeding, with about 3–5 sucks per swallow before milk is in, and 1–2 times per swallow afterward.[1]
- ❏ Is easy to keep awake during the 20- to 30-minute feeding.
- ❏ Shows no more than 75th percentile weight loss on the NEWT.
- ❏ Shows no more than 7 percent weight loss from birth weight.
- ❏ Has moist lips and mouth.
- ❏ Has hydrated skin that doesn't stay wrinkled when gently squeezed.
- ❏ Has a flat soft spot (fontanelle).
- ❏ Has minimal yellowing of skin, limited to the face and white of the eyes.
- ❏ Has clear or light yellow urine.
- ❏ Has 6–8 wet diapers and 3 or more dirty diapers a day once they are getting full feedings. (Note: For exclusively breastfed newborns, diapers counts are unreliable until milk comes in.)

Blood Markers of a Well-Fed Newborn

Glucose[2]	>50 mg/dL in first 48 hours >60 mg/dL after 48 hours
Sodium[3]	135–145 mEq/L
Total Bilirubin[4]	<13.5 mg/dL (safest for brain development)

Signs of a Hungry Newborn

H	Hypoglycemia (low blood sugar), characterized by jittery hands, low body temperature, inconsolable and high-pitched crying, lethargy, limpness, turning blue, and seizures
U	Unsatisfied nursing, lasting longer than 30 minutes and occurring more frequently than every 2 hours; crying despite prolonged breastfeeding
N	Not waking for feeding every 3 hours, nodding off during feeds, difficult to arouse, not maintaining latch, limp, lethargic
G	Growth is poor—weight loss exceeds 7%, weight gain is less than 6 oz/week (170 grams/week) once newborn starts gaining
R	Reduced wet and dirty diaper counts (no wet diapers in 6 hours), red-orange "brick dust" in diapers, dry lips and mouth, skin that wrinkles
Y	Yellowing of the eyes or skin, especially below the face (excessive jaundice)

ESTIMATED NEWBORN MILK INTAKE

As described in chapter four, newborns experience a recovery period for several hours after birth where they often take in less than their full milk requirement. Eventually, however, they become hungry for their full requirement. The table at the top of page 152 provides an estimate of this.

Remember, every newborn is born with different caloric and fluid reserves, and so some tolerate a short period of underfeeding better than others. Some will need more than the volumes in the chart on page 152; some will need less. Most babies are able to avoid unsafe conditions if given access to the milk they are hungry for.

Average Term Newborn Human Milk or Formula Intake per Feed, if Fed to Satisfaction[5]

Time After Birth	Volume per Feed (oz)		Volume per Feed for an Average (3.2 kg/ 7 lb) Baby, If Given Every 3 Hours
	Per lb	Per kg	
Postbirth recovery period (0–24 hours after birth)*	0.15	0.35	0.5–1 oz
When baby becomes hungry for full feedings (after the recovery period)	0.3	0.7	2.2 oz

*Based on the known term newborn resting energy requirement of 50 calories/kg/day, which approximates the minimum number of calories required to maintain basic vital functions.[6] The duration of the recovery period varies among babies.

We recommend that every parent calculate their newborn's estimated daily calorie and milk requirement based on their birth weight to know what they need after the recovery period. You can do this using the chart below, or the Fed Is Best Daily Milk Calculator, available at the QR code below the chart. This should serve *only* as an estimate of what a term newborn needs once they are hungry for their full nutritional requirement; the true amount may be slightly more or less than this average, depending on their hunger and satisfaction cues. Parents whose children developed feeding complications commonly report *never* being told in their educational resources or by their health professionals how much milk their baby needed to be adequately fed.

Average Daily Caloric Requirement of Newborn Infants (0–1 Month)	
Full daily caloric requirement[7]	110 calories/kg of infant body weight/day* (range: 100–120 cal/kg/day)
Mature breast milk or formula requirement to meet caloric requirement	5.5 oz/kg/day or 2.5 oz/lb/day Note: Average mature breast milk and standard formula have 20 cal/oz, although the caloric content of breast milk varies.[8]
Full daily milk requirement of newborns by weight[9]	5.5 oz/kg/day × _____ kg = _____ oz milk/day 2.5 oz/lb/day × _____ lb = _____ oz milk/day
Number of feeds per day	8–10
Ounces per feed**	_____ total oz milk/day ÷ # of feeds = _____ oz milk/feed (usually 1.5–3 oz per feed to satisfaction)[10]
Example for 7 lb baby**	7 lb × 2.5 oz/lb/day = 17.5 oz/day 17.5 oz/day ÷ 8 feeds/day = 2.2 oz feed (on average)

*The calories that most nutritional labels refer to, scientifically, are actually kilocalories. We recommend using kilograms (kg) to calculate caloric requirements, as using pounds and ounces of weight (lb, oz) can lead to errors. Scan the QR code to go to the Fed Is Best Daily Milk Calculator to calculate your infant's average daily milk requirement.

**The amount per feed can fluctuate throughout the day and the intervals between feeds can vary.

FED IS BEST GUIDELINES FOR SUFFICIENT NEWBORN BREASTFEEDING

If you're planning to breastfeed, it's important not only to learn how to latch but also to ensure your baby is effectively removing and drinking milk. To help you do this, we have developed guidelines to get breastfeeding off to the best possible start while ensuring sufficient feeding.

1. Do skin-to-skin and breastfeed within the first hour or as soon as possible once mother and baby are stable, with close monitoring and guidance from a qualified health professional. Clinical trials have shown this to promote sustained breastfeeding (see page 178 for details).

2. Check for the presence of colostrum by manual expression before *every* feeding; some nursing moms have scant to no colostrum, particularly on the second day.[11]

3. Get help with breastfeeding technique to ensure good latch and milk transfer. Ineffective breastfeeding can impair milk production and colostrum intake.

4. Ensure adequate time effectively nursing on each breast for at least 10–15 minutes every 2–3 hours, in response to your baby's hunger signs.

5. If your baby is not nursing effectively, hand-express breasts or pump for 10–15 minutes with a double electric pump to ensure adequate stimulation and maximal colostrum/milk removal.

6. Feed all your expressed breast milk. If it is greater than 15 mL (0.5 oz), you can pause for a few seconds to check for continued hunger signs, then continue feeding.

7. If supplementation is needed, offer 15 mL of banked donor milk and/or formula, but only after adequate nursing. Repeat supplementation according to hunger cues. (See more about supplementing on page 157.)

SECOND NIGHT SYNDROME IN EXCLUSIVELY BREASTFED BABIES: IS IT A SIGN OF INADEQUATE FEEDING?

On the second day after birth, many exclusively breastfed babies may seem really hungry. They want to breastfeed all day and all night but don't appear satisfied, even after an extended feeding session. As soon as they are finished, they may cry and want to breastfeed again. Parents are often told that this behavior is *normal and necessary* to bring in the full milk supply and that their baby is not really hungry.[12]

There is no evidence that newborns need to feed longer than thirty minutes or more frequently than twelve times a day to promote onset of lactogenesis II or higher milk production. Indeed, full milk comes in for most mothers whether or not their infant breastfeeds at all.[13] Furthermore, scientific evidence shows that exclusively breastfed newborns on the second day are, in fact, hungry *and* thirsty, as reflected by markers of relative fasting during this period, namely declining glucose levels, rising ketones and sodium levels, and weight loss (see the section beginning on page 42).[14]

Babies who are getting enough milk sleep contentedly between feedings. If your baby is constantly or frantically crying and nursing, they are telling you they are hungry. *Do not let anyone talk you out of listening to your baby.*

> On my baby's second day, he had to take his hearing test multiple times because he wouldn't stop screaming; we couldn't get newborn photos because he wouldn't stop screaming; we couldn't walk down to the breastfeeding class because he wouldn't stop screaming . . . The grandmas wanted desperately to give a pacifier and help feed him, but it had only taken 48 hours in the hospital and the raw fear of new motherhood to turn me into an avid exclusive breastfeeder. They said I should do this so I have to do this. I follow the rules, I do what is best, I am a doctor, I have to do this, they said I had to . . . It had now been five days since I last slept. [T]he lab test resulted in immediate readmission for bili lights [phototherapy]. His total bilirubin was 21—a number that I will never forget . . . If only I had had the capacity to use my doctor brain then, but I simply couldn't. I was just trying to survive.
>
> —Nicole King, MD

WHEN TO SEEK PROFESSIONAL
EVALUATION FOR FEEDING

Whether you are at the hospital or at home, do not hesitate to get help if you feel feeding is not going well, to make sure that your baby is getting the nutrition they need and that, if you are breastfeeding, you are doing so effectively.

If breastfeeding, get assistance for the following:

1. If your baby's latch is poor, shallow, or painful, or positioning is uncomfortable, have a lactation professional evaluate your breastfeeding technique.

2. If you are concerned about your newborn being persistently hungry (see the HUNGRY infographic on page 151), have your baby weighed and plotted on the NEWT and evaluated by a physician. If there is weight loss at or above the 75th percentile or greater than 7 percent, we recommend feeding technique evaluation and having blood work like glucose, bilirubin, and sodium done. If your baby has been fed all your available milk and there is a delay in getting an evaluation, supplement to alleviate your baby's hunger until the evaluation can be done.

3. If your baby is showing visible signs of low blood sugar, excessive jaundice, or dehydration, have their blood glucose, bilirubin, and electrolytes checked immediately. If they have been fed all your available milk, offer supplementation while waiting for results—these conditions are unsafe to leave uncorrected while waiting, should they turn out to be abnormal.

4. If weight loss and lab values are borderline or abnormal, supplement *to satisfaction* with mother's expressed breast milk, banked donor milk, or formula to treat or prevent further escalation of feeding complications. Some cases may require additional medical treatment by a pediatrician or neonatologist.

5. If clinical evaluation, laboratory testing, and/or infant weighing are not immediately available (if, for example, you are already at

home) and you have concerns about your child being persistently hungry despite breastfeeding, check for the presence of ample milk with expression and honor your baby's hunger cues. **If you have *any* doubts, the safest thing to do is to err on the side of caution and supplement in 15 mL increments after nursing.** Repeat as needed until your baby is satisfied. This will prevent any escalation of feeding complications until your milk comes in. Then pump or hand-express colostrum to protect your milk supply.

Problems of inadequate feeding that result in an inconsolable baby commonly occur between discharge and the baby's follow-up visit if full milk has not come in. You can supplement while arranging an urgent appointment with your baby's physician. Most pediatric clinics have an after-hours nurse line as well. **Make sure you state that feeding your baby enough is more important to you than avoiding supplementation.** Again, it is better to err on the side of caution by feeding your baby than risk their developing a medical problem that results in a hospital admission, or worse.

While some parents are advised not to have formula in the house to "avoid temptation," in many of the stories we have received, this advice has led to frantic late-night trips to the store for formula, which parents did not know how to choose or prepare, ultimately contributing to a readmission for feeding complications.

HOW TO SUPPLEMENT BREASTFEEDING IF NEEDED

If your baby needs supplemental milk, the most important element of maintaining your milk supply is frequent and effective removal of milk. **Failure to adequately and frequently remove milk can signal the body to reduce milk production, resulting in lower milk supply and/or breastfeeding cessation, a condition called secondary lactation failure.** This does not mean that if you miss one breastfeeding or pumping session, your milk supply will instantly disappear; only if poor milk removal is sustained does this happen.

Parents are commonly taught that supplementation is the *cause* of secondary lactation failure when it is actually ineffective and/or infrequent breastfeeding, inadequate milk removal, or both that reduce milk production. If supplemental milk (either banked human milk or formula) is offered *before* breastfeeding, the baby may be satisfied before the breasts are maximally drained, which can reduce milk production and increase the need for supplemental milk. If supplemental milk is offered after effective nursing or pumping, then the stimulus for milk production should be maintained.

Parents are also taught that a baby given supplemental formula will not be hungry enough to breastfeed, resulting in a downward spiral of milk production. Newborns are hungry around every three hours regardless of how they are fed. So, there is ample opportunity for them to nurse directly and learn to latch effectively. Remember, supplemented breastfeeding has been the most common form of breastfeeding across the globe for millennia prior to the BFHI era, especially in the first days after birth.

Step-by-Step Guide to Supplementing a Breastfed Newborn While Maintaining Milk Production and Latching

1. Follow the Fed Is Best Guidelines for Sufficient Newborn Feeding on page 153.
2. If nursing is ineffective, express milk manually or with a pump and feed it to your baby with a syringe.
3. If your baby is still hungry, further supplementation can be done with banked donor milk or formula through one of the following methods:
   a. 15 mL at a time with a curved-tip syringe slipped into the corner of your baby's mouth while latched at the breast.
   b. 15 mL at a time with a supplemental nursing system (see page 141) while the baby is latched at the breast.
   c. 15 mL at a time with a bottle and slow-flow nipple.
   (Note: 5–7 mL feeds have *not* been shown to be effective at reversing feeding complications.)

4. Pause and burp baby after each supplemental feeding and observe for signs of continued hunger.

5. Repeat steps 3 and 4 until your baby is satisfied.

6. Continue supplementation of feedings until your milk supply meets your baby's requirement and any other indications for supplementation are resolved.

ONSET OF LACTOGENESIS II AND MANAGING ENGORGEMENT

Ideally, the onset of lactogenesis II for breastfeeding parents, when milk production increases rapidly, comes roughly between thirty-six and seventy-two hours after birth, before the baby loses more weight than they can safely tolerate (which sometimes occurs before seventy-two hours). You may notice your breasts feel fuller, tender, or warm to the touch; this signals the onset of lactogenesis II, when colostrum begins to transition into mature milk. The yellowish color of colostrum should gradually become lighter and increase in volume. A full milk supply is initially greater than an infant's full requirement, providing a healthy cushion of excess milk. You may experience a "letdown" sensation when your baby's suckling causes the breast to release its stored milk to satisfy your infant (don't worry if you don't feel this; not everyone does). Learn more about lactogenesis II by scanning the QR code.

This rapid increase in milk production can result in severe engorgement, which can narrow the milk ducts and reduce flow. Over time, unrelieved engorgement, called **milk stasis,** can reduce milk production. During this initial engorgement phase, which usually lasts about two to three days, make sure to remove milk from your breasts regularly by nursing or pumping to avoid milk stasis. Your breasts should be noticeably softer after nursing if your baby is transferring milk well.

The first fourteen days are a critical time for your supply to be established. A full supply is typically 25–27 ounces of milk per day by day 14, increasing to 29 ounces or more by six months—enough for your baby to maintain their growth curve.[15] Regular nursing or pumping and managing engorgement are key to supporting the production of enough milk to fully feed your baby. It is also important for avoiding mastitis and/or a breast abscess, infections that require antibiotic treatment and sometimes surgical drainage, and can result in a reduction in milk supply as well.[16]

MANAGING ENGORGEMENT THAT PREVENTS EFFECTIVE FEEDING

If you develop engorgement that changes your nipple shape so much that it prevents latching and effective milk transfer, or it prevents you from having milk letdown, try the following:

1. Cold compresses to the breasts between feeding sessions and anti-inflammatory medication may help reduce swelling.[17]
2. Try nursing in a laid-back position.
3. Use **reverse pressure softening** (providing gentle pressure with fingertips on the areola for about a minute or two before nursing or pumping).[18]
4. Hand-express or pump for just a few minutes to relieve the fullness, then try latching.
5. If none of these things work, a temporary nipple shield might help; after the breast has softened, remove the shield and latch back onto the breast.

Whatever happens, there is no need to panic. You can pump your breasts, give your baby expressed milk, and try again at the next feeding.[19]

RISK FACTORS FOR INSUFFICIENT FEEDING

As we have discussed, feeding problems are very common in the first few days. While some problems arise from ineffective breastfeeding technique, which can be corrected, others stem from things that are out of your control. Therefore, it is important to have a plan to handle these challenges so that you and your baby can have the best possible experience and outcomes.

Delayed Lactogenesis II

When lactogenesis II doesn't occur within seventy-two hours of birth, it's referred to as delayed lactogenesis II (DLII). Last chapter, we discussed DLII as one of the most common feeding challenges for breastfeeding parents. It's also an obvious risk factor for insufficient feeding and a common indication for supplementation. Remember, research shows that before milk comes in, exclusively breastfed newborns are experiencing a state of underfeeding, as evidenced by declining blood sugar levels (glucose), rising ketone and sodium levels (markers of hunger and dehydration), and weight loss.[20] If full milk supply does not arrive before a baby's caloric and fluid reserves run out, and the baby is not supplemented, the baby will experience unsafe glucose and sodium levels. Some infants may not be able to wait seventy-two hours to get their full milk requirement and need supplementation earlier. Research has also shown that delayed lactogenesis II is a risk factor for early cessation of breastfeeding.[21]

Several factors affect the onset of full milk production: adequate frequency and time nursing, effective milk removal, physical stress around delivery, and the risk factors discussed starting on page 133. Some of these can be modified with lactation management and tools; others cannot.

For mothers at risk for DLII due to ineffective feeding:

1. Make sure to correct any problems with latch and milk transfer with the help of a lactation professional, as impaired milk removal can delay lactogenesis II.

   2. If your baby is feeding ineffectively even with professional help,
   pumping at least every three hours (to replace ineffective feeding
   sessions) can still provide the stimulus to produce milk. In fact, a
   clinical trial has found that **fifteen minutes of pumping with a
   double electric pump *at least* six times a day, including once
   at night, starting within an hour of birth, along with direct
   breastfeeding**, helped milk come in more quickly on average
   (three days versus four days) and increased the average milk volume
   on day 3 (74 mL vs. 25 mL) and on day 7 (225 mL vs. 69 mL).[22]

The most frequent recommendation for addressing delayed
lactogenesis II is a regimen of breastfeeding, pumping, *and* supplementing,
also called triple feeding (see page 196 for more on triple feeding). Once
milk supply meets a baby's full requirement and sufficient milk transfer
is confirmed, this regimen can be stopped. Note that this triple-feeding
regimen should only be done for a week *at most*, as it can cause severe sleep
deprivation, impair parents, and compromise infant safety. During that
week, a partner or family member should help with baby care and keeping
the feeding equipment clean, to reduce stress on the breastfeeding parent.

   **Ultimately, the earlier and more frequently breast milk is removed,
the quicker the milk comes in and the greater the quantity within
your breasts' potential.** However, you must balance hand expression and
pumping with the need to be gentle with your nipples and the need for sleep
and recovery.

STRESSES AROUND DELIVERY THAT
DELAY LACTOGENESIS II

Delivering a baby is one of the most physically stressful events of a
woman's life. Multiple markers of stress have been associated with
delayed onset of lactogenesis II and lower milk production once
it comes in.[23] Among the conditions that tend to cause maternal

stress are cesarean sections and prolonged or complicated vaginal deliveries.

In the United States, as well as other countries, a third of all deliveries are cesarean sections.[24] For mothers who deliver by cesarean section, particularly if it is urgent, the stress of a surgical delivery may cause high cortisol levels that lead to DLII.[25] It is not uncommon for first-time mothers of babies delivered by cesarean section to have their milk come in at day 6 or 7.

Similarly, mothers who have prolonged, stressful, or complicated vaginal deliveries, like vacuum delivery or excessive blood loss (>500 mL), have higher rates of DLII.[26] In fact, more severe blood loss (>1,500 mL) can even result in failed lactogenesis II,[27] where milk does not come in at all. If you experience a prolonged or complicated delivery, you will need to work daily with your lactation consultant to ensure you are effectively nursing or pumping with minimal pain.

Baby Born Premature (35–37 Weeks), Late Preterm (37–38 Weeks), or Small for Gestational Age

Early (<38 weeks) and small-for-gestational-age babies (SGA, or <10th percentile weight for gestational age) have fewer calorie and fluid reserves, and thus are more vulnerable to not getting enough milk.* They are also much sleepier than term average-size babies, and thus are less likely to (a) remove milk effectively, or (b) stimulate the breasts vigorously enough to make more milk. For these reasons, they are at greater risk for low blood sugar

---

* Small-for-gestational-age babies are small because they had a poorly functioning placenta that prevented them from getting all the nutrients they needed. Therefore, even if an SGA baby is full term, they, like premature babies, often have low caloric reserves, are less able to tolerate underfeeding, and don't breastfeed as vigorously as full-term average-size babies.

(hypoglycemia), require glucose monitoring, and often need earlier supplementation to treat hypoglycemia.

For mothers of early and/or SGA babies, pumping is often added to the feeding plan to maximize stimulation for milk production in the critical first weeks. Supplementation is also used to give these babies the energy to breastfeed more effectively. Sometimes this is done with oral dextrose (glucose) gel, which trials show is effective at reducing hypoglycemia.[28] But research shows that giving oral dextrose *with* formula or banked donor milk is more effective at stabilizing blood glucose than giving oral dextrose alone.[29] Since these babies have a greater risk of breastfeeding not working out, it's important to get help early if you are having problems.

Baby Born Large for Gestational Age or to a Diabetic Mother

Larger babies and babies of diabetic mothers (often born large) have higher caloric needs due to higher body weight. Infants of diabetic mothers also have high circulating insulin levels that can lower blood glucose. If either type of baby doesn't receive adequate calories through feeding, they are prone to unsafe low glucose levels. Like early and SGA babies, they require glucose monitoring and commonly need supplementation.

These babies are often less patient during feedings because their high caloric requirements make them hungrier. If they are frantic with hunger and refusing to latch, they often benefit from an "appetizer" of 5–10 mL of expressed breast milk or formula before going to breast. This can be done with a curved-tip syringe at the breast or a bottle.

DISCHARGE PLANNING AND MONITORING WEIGHT AFTER DISCHARGE

Having a discharge plan to monitor and ensure adequate feeding is important for avoiding feeding complications at home. Most healthy, term, vaginally delivered US newborns are discharged at thirty-six to forty-eight hours or less, while cesarean-delivered newborns are usually discharged before seventy-two hours. Ideally, infants should get a weight check immediately before discharge. In some hospitals, the last weight check is at midnight before discharge, which can be twelve or more hours before patients leave, during which the baby is likely still losing weight. Many infants who have required readmission have had marginal weight loss of 7–8 percent measured hours prior to discharge; their feeding problems could have been diagnosed if their weight had been rechecked just prior to discharge.

Research shows that the risk of feeding complications begins to increase at 7–8 percent weight loss.[30] Separate studies also have shown that the two to three days after birth—often the time between discharge and the first follow-up appointment—are typically when the greatest weight loss occurs and are when the risk of developing feeding complications is highest.[31] Accordingly, we recommend that all exclusively breast-fed infants, especially those with 7 percent weight loss or greater, or who are at or higher than the 75th percentile on the NEWT before discharge, get laboratory screening of glucose, sodium, and/or bilirubin to determine if it is safe to discharge them. If milk has not yet come in, then the weight loss should be expected to continue, and a plan for supplementation should be provided.

USING A HOME BABY SCALE TO MONITOR WEIGHT

You can use a home baby scale to monitor your newborn's weight every twelve hours until your milk comes in, then enter this data into the NEWT at www.newbornweight.org.[32] If your baby loses more than 7 percent of their birth weight or is higher than 75th percentile on the NEWT, whichever occurs first, and/or they have HUNGRY signs (see page 151), you can supplement to satisfaction after nursing while you make an appointment to promptly see their health provider. It is important to err on the side of caution, as you don't have the means to diagnose feeding complications at home.

If you are exclusively breastfeeding and your baby is still losing weight at discharge, you should make a next-day pediatrician appointment. If you are being discharged on Friday and weekend appointments are unavailable, your baby's doctor should offer guidance on appropriate supplementation if your milk comes in late or your baby is still showing signs of hunger after breastfeeding.

If you are not sure if your milk has come in, you can manually express or pump your breasts for one feed to estimate how much your baby is receiving. If you can only express a few milliliters, your milk is not in, and supplementation is needed. If you can pump about 30–60 mL per feed, your milk is likely coming in. Feed your baby your expressed milk, then breastfeed at least every three hours. (Note that while some mothers may have difficulty at first in responding to a pump, most find that pumping provides a good estimate of the available milk.)[33]

CHECKLIST FOR SAFE DISCHARGE OF AN EXCLUSIVELY BREASTFED NEWBORN

- Has your baby been calm and satisfied with most feeds?
- Is percentage weight loss less than 7 percent and less than the 75th percentile on the NEWT?
- Are bilirubin levels below 13.5 mg/dL?
- Are glucose levels normal (>50 mg/dL before 48 hours, >60 mg/dL after 48 hours)?
- If weight loss is greater than 7 percent, or the baby is unsatisfied with feeding at 5–7 percent, are sodium levels normal?

Newborns with borderline or abnormal weight loss or bilirubin, sodium, or glucose values may require extended admission or a next-day clinic visit with a supplementation plan. Newborns with reassuring feeding behavior and feeding-related data, and whose mothers' full milk supply is in, can be followed up forty-eight to seventy-two hours after discharge.

FIRST PEDIATRIC VISIT

All newborns get a follow-up appointment, usually one to three days after discharge from their health facility. If your baby is continuing to lose weight because your milk is not in at the time of discharge, your baby's first follow-up visit should be the next day. One of the purposes of this visit is to evaluate how well they are feeding and their percentage weight loss.

There are a few important questions to ask your baby's doctor during this check-up:

- What is my baby's percentage weight loss and what does the NEWT curve look like?
- Is my baby jaundiced? If so, what is their bilirubin level and where does it fall on the bilirubin nomogram (the graph that physicians use to determine the need for phototherapy)? Does it require phototherapy and/or a supplementation plan?
- Are there signs of dehydration? If the weight loss is more than 7 percent, will we check for hypernatremia?
- Are there signs of low blood sugar? If so, can we check their glucose level?

Your baby's doctor is your advisor and partner in protecting your baby's health. Don't be afraid to communicate honestly about your concerns and to ask for objective data to provide you reassurance that your baby is getting enough nutrition.

Multiple studies have shown that the leading causes of readmission for healthy term newborns are for preventable insufficient feeding complications, like high sodium, dehydration, and jaundice, which occur more commonly to exclusively breastfed newborns who lose greater than 7 percent of their birth weight.[34] If your baby has greater than 7 percent weight loss and/or has signs of persistent hunger, a basic metabolic panel and bilirubin test can diagnose low blood sugar, hyperbilirubinemia, and hypernatremic dehydration. Laboratory data is important to accurately diagnose and safely correct the subset of feeding complications that cannot be identified by clinical exam. Start supplemental feeding while waiting for results.

If you are exclusively breastfeeding, your baby is continuing to lose weight, and your milk is not in at this appointment, ask for guidance on supplementation and for another next-day follow-up appointment. Continue to follow their weight every twelve hours at home or get a weight check at the clinic until they start gaining weight.

If your milk is in but you have concerns about adequate transfer of milk during breastfeeding, ask for an evaluation by a lactation consultant and a weighted feed. A weighted feed is done by weighing a baby on a scale accurate to ±2 g before and after a breastfeeding session and measuring the difference. Your baby should be receiving around 0.3 fluid ounces per pound or 0.7 fluid ounces per kilogram each feeding session (around 2–3 oz per feed for a full-term, average-weight baby) if feeding every three hours.

If your baby's weight check and exam are normal and your milk is in, continue to follow your baby's hunger cues and nurse every two to three hours on demand. If your baby is sleepy, it's important to wake them at least every three hours to feed until they begin waking on their own for feeding. If there are concerns about feeding, continue to work with your baby's doctor and your lactation consultant and follow our supplementation guide (see page 157) to maintain your milk supply. Once they are getting their full milk requirement, your baby should be gaining about 0.9 to 1.1 ounces per day (26 to 34 grams per day) or six to eight ounces per week (180 to 240 grams per week) and following their growth curve on the CDC or WHO growth chart, which we discuss more on page 190.

AT THE END OF THE DAY, FEEDING IS THE FIRST PRIORITY

Adequate feeding is the foundation of optimal infant feeding. Especially if you are exclusively breastfeeding, ensuring adequate feeding requires careful monitoring of feeding efficacy, infant weight, and, at times, blood work. Most of all, it requires careful attention to your baby's signs of hunger and satisfaction. If your baby is showing signs of persistent hunger and distress despite feeding, get a full evaluation of your baby's nutritional status from their doctor, with percentage weight loss data and blood work, and of your breastfeeding technique from your lactation professional. Supplement your baby for persistent hunger and for any signs of feeding complications, especially if there is any delay in getting an evaluation or lab results. If your baby stops crying with supplementation, then you know what the problem was. You can work on fixing the problem without your baby suffering.

Ultimately, receiving adequate nutrition, whether with breast milk, formula, or both, is the best way to ensure optimal health outcomes for your baby. These will look different for every family. Just listen to your baby. They will tell you what they need.

7

Breastfeeding

Most mothers start out wanting to breastfeed. Yet, for multiple reasons, breastfeeding rates drop off sharply and continue falling over the first six months of a baby's life. According to the 2022 CDC Breastfeeding Report Card, 83.2 percent of US mothers initiate breastfeeding, with 56 percent continuing to breastfeed and 25 percent exclusively breastfeeding at six months.[1] Globally, 68 percent of children are breastfeeding at one year and 44 percent at 2 years, with 44 percent exclusively breastfeeding at six months.[2]

Most mothers want to breastfeed because multiple health organizations recommend exclusive breastfeeding (EBF) due to observational studies showing multiple health advantages in breastfed babies, including reduced rates of respiratory and gastrointestinal infections, allergic diseases, and obesity, among other benefits (although some advantages may be related to parental and household factors associated with breastfeeding; see chapter three). Other reasons why parents choose EBF include:

- possible health benefits to mother, like lower rates of diabetes; hypertension; and breast, ovarian, and endometrial cancer[3] (although it is unclear if breastfeeding causes better maternal health or if healthier mothers are more able or likely to breastfeed).
- enjoyment of breastfeeding and feeling of closeness to one's baby.
- the convenience of having a ready source of healthy nutrition for their baby.
- the cost of formula.
- family or cultural tradition.
- personal preference.

Breastfeeding is defined as providing human milk to a baby directly at the breast or by alternative feeding methods (e.g., bottles). *Successful* breastfeeding means that *both* people in the breastfeeding relationship are thriving physically and mentally. For mothers with ample colostrum, timely onset of a full milk supply, and effective latch, EBF is a desirable and healthy option. For those with transiently low milk supply, temporary supplementation may be needed. For others with persistent low milk supply, combination feeding may be needed. *All* of these can be considered successful breastfeeding. Your success isn't determined by the number of ounces you produce, but rather by whether your baby, you, and your family are happy and healthy as a result of your unique breastfeeding relationship.

Successful breastfeeding is also *safe* breastfeeding—breastfeeding that prioritizes preventing infant hunger and thirst as well as complications caused by inadequate feeding *over* breastfeeding exclusivity. The most important goals of feeding a baby are to provide (1) an uncontaminated and nutritionally complete source of nutrition, and (2) a *sufficient quantity* of nutrition to provide all a baby needs to live and grow. Both are necessary to optimize an infant's health and future development.

During your breastfeeding journey, it is important to always keep in mind the reason you wanted to breastfeed in the first place. Why? Parents

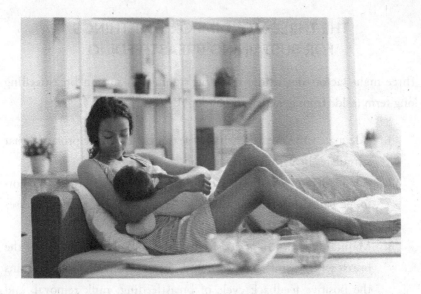

who experienced severe problems have told us that they persisted in breast-feeding even after their reasons for breastfeeding—bonding, infant health, saving money—were not materializing or were working against what they wanted (for example, they were spending more time with their pump than their baby or their infant was failing to gain weight).

There are many products and recommendations out there for sustaining breastfeeding and increasing milk supply. Some have moderate benefits. Many are either ineffective or have weak data supporting their usefulness. The first part of this chapter reviews how effective these different methods are in promoting breastfeeding, to help you decide what is worth trying. The rest of the chapter teaches how to manage breastfeeding once it has been established.

I loved nursing my daughters for the convenience and the close-ness it provided. It felt magical that I could both nourish and soothe my babies from my own body.

—Jayne Freeman

THE THREE MOST IMPORTANT THINGS
FOR SUSTAINING BREASTFEEDING

Three main factors determine a mother's ability to sustain breastfeeding long term (aside from genetics and biology):

1. Adequate time nursing, which releases the hormone prolactin that stimulates breast milk production.[4]
2. Adequate removal of milk from the breasts, which reduces the hormone called feedback inhibitor of lactation (FIL) that suppresses milk production.[5]
3. Maintaining an infant's desire to nurse directly by associating the breast with warmth, comfort, and/or nourishment, which sustains the positive feedback cycle of breastfeeding, milk removal, and milk production.

Even when supplementation is needed, due to low milk supply or delayed onset of full milk production, it does not mean your chances of sustaining breastfeeding are ruined. The key is to introduce supplementation in a way that does not interfere with this positive feedback cycle, namely by (1) offering supplements after ensuring frequent and adequate milk transfer to your baby during nursing; (2) removing milk with a pump; and (3) feeding in response to hunger cues, stopping when your baby is satisfied (see page 153).

In addition, *your* experience of breastfeeding is one of the foundations of making it work long term. Acknowledging how breastfeeding makes you feel, and *honoring* those feelings by adjusting your breastfeeding regimen so that it is healthy for *you*, is also important.

THE WHO TEN STEPS TO SUCCESSFUL
BREASTFEEDING: HOW HELPFUL ARE THEY?

Breastfeeding is typically promoted using the WHO Ten Steps to Successful Breastfeeding (see page 28).[6] It's currently the method through which breastfeeding is promoted in hospitals under the Baby-Friendly Hospital Initiative (BFHI). While any program that teaches families how to initiate breastfeeding, as the Ten Steps does, is expected to improve breastfeeding rates, not *all* of the Ten Steps improve breastfeeding equally—in fact, some have no effect at all.

The largest clinical trial on the Ten Steps and the BFHI was done in Belarus in the mid-1990s, called the Promotion of Breastfeeding Intervention Trial, or PROBIT, which randomly assigned hospitals to receive breastfeeding promotion intervention or standard care. Breast-feeding rates in Belarus in the 1990s were low, with the earliest data (2005) showing breastfeeding rates at twelve to twenty-three months of 12.6 percent and EBF rates of 10.3 percent. The outcomes showed the BFHI was effective at increasing rates of breastfeeding to any degree (called "any breastfeeding") with 12 percent higher rates at three months, 13.7 percent higher rates at six months, 11.7 percent higher rates at nine months, and 8.3 percent higher rates at twelve months. EBF was a new standard, so those in the intervention group were much more likely to be exclusively breastfeeding at three months (43.3% vs. 6.4%) and at six months (7.9% vs. 0.6%).

However, more recent data on the BFHI in the US does not show as strong an effect. A 2019 study looked at the effect of having a higher per-centage of births occurring at BFHI-certified hospitals in all fifty states on "postdischarge breastfeeding rates," namely rates of EBF at three and six months and any breastfeeding at six and twelve months. It found that states with more births at BFHI hospitals did not correlate with higher postdischarge breastfeeding rates. What did correlate with higher breastfeeding rates were higher breastfeeding *initiation* rates. But were breastfeeding initiation rates higher in states with more BFHI births? No. The authors concluded that helping families initiate breastfeeding was more effective at promoting sustained breastfeeding than hospital BFHI certification. A similar opinion was made by the US Preventive Task Services Force, which reviewed data on breastfeeding promotion and concluded that, while individual-level breastfeeding counseling was effective at increasing breastfeeding rates, system-level programs like the BFHI were not.[7]

Regardless, there *are* key interventions that help families initiate and sustain breastfeeding, including a few of the Ten Steps. In 2017, the WHO gathered an expert panel to systematically review the highest-quality data on the individual steps to assess how effective they were at promoting breastfeeding and to assess their risks in order to determine which steps to retain.[8] It would surprise most people to learn that only two and a half (the half being "give no water") of the Ten Steps have been shown to improve breastfeeding rates. And the most widely recommended step, Step 6, "Give newborn infants no food or drink other than breast milk, unless medically indicated," referring to avoiding formula, was the *least effective* of the Ten Steps in promoting breastfeeding, with data showing judicious supplementation actually *improved* breastfeeding rates. Despite this data, the WHO continues to recommend it.

For a detailed summary of the WHO expert panel's assessment of the Ten Steps, scan the QR code. We have summarized the findings most relevant to parents, with our own recommendations on modifying the Ten Steps in italics, below, to give you an idea how beneficial (or not) they are and what the risks are, if any, so that you can decide how much importance to give each step.

The Most Helpful Steps

1. Parent education on breastfeeding before and around the time of birth (Step 3).
   a. Improves any BF and EBF at 6 months by 11 percent.
   b. Improves any BF at 4–6 weeks by 12 percent.
   c. Improves EBF at 4–6 weeks by 21 percent.
2. Skin-to-skin care within the first 23 hours if mom and baby are stable (part 1 of Step 4).
   a. Improves BF at discharge to 1 month by 30 percent.
   b. Improves EBF at 6 weeks to 6 months by 50 percent.
   c. Improves any BF at 1–4 months by 24 percent.

Note: It did not matter whether skin-to-skin contact was done immediately (within ten minutes of birth) or within the first twenty-three hours. Skin-to-skin care (SSC) was also associated with increased risks of infant suffocation and falling from bed if the parent falls asleep during SSC, but this risk can be reduced with close health professional supervision.

3. Early initiation of breastfeeding within the first hour if mother and baby are medically stable, with close supervision similar to SSC (part 2 of Step 4).
    a. When compared to initiation between 1 hour and 23 hours:
        i.   Increases EBF rates at 1 month by 15 percent.
        ii. Increases EBF rates at 3 months by 5 percent.
    b. When compared to initiation after 24 hours:
        i.   Increases EBF rates at 1 month by 24 percent.
        ii. Increases EBF at 3 months by 6 percent.
4. Giving no additional water (which applies to all infants until solid food is introduced) (part 2 of Step 6).
    a. Increases any BF at 4 weeks by 17 percent.
    b. Increases any BF at 12 weeks by 32 percent.
    c. Increases any BF at 20 weeks by 31 percent.

Steps That Have Little to No Benefit or Are Counterproductive to Sustained Breastfeeding, and/or Are Potentially Harmful

1. Giving no additional food (like formula) other than breast milk unless medically indicated (part 1 of Step 6) is *counterproductive*, but retained by the WHO panel.
    a. Judicious supplementation improved breastfeeding rates by 20 percent at 3 months.
    b. Judicious supplementation improved EBF rates by 43 percent at 3 months.
    Note: With the addition of three later studies not included in the initial review, it seems likely judicious supplementation has no significant effect on breastfeeding rates.

2. Rooming in 24/7 (Step 7) improved breastfeeding rates at day 4 after birth by 92 percent but had no significant effect on sustained breastfeeding at 3–4 or 6 months. *Nursery care may be needed for parents who are exhausted, medicated, or in pain due to the risk of maternal exhaustion, accidental bed sharing, and infant suffocation.*

3. Avoidance of pacifiers and bottles (Step 9) had no effects on breastfeeding rates and is potentially harmful since pacifiers reduce the risk of SIDS.

GETTING BREASTFEEDING OFF TO A GOOD START

Getting the best start to breastfeeding requires preparation, knowledge of breastfeeding technique and management, recognition of infant hunger and satisfaction cues, and most of all, flexibility. Much of this is covered in chapters five and six, and in our online resources linked there and later in this chapter, but the following are recommendations that have been shown in clinical trials to be beneficial to sustaining breastfeeding.

Skin-to-Skin Care

SSC has been shown to be associated with moderate increases in exclusive and any breastfeeding up to six months.[9] The transition to life outside the uterus can be stressful; SSC can help stabilize the baby's body temperature and heart rate, reduce crying, and stabilize their blood sugar by slowing down how fast they burn calories to stay warm, while they get to know you during this special time.[10] (Note that SSC alone is not enough to *correct* low blood sugar, which requires giving glucose by mouth or intravenously, or feeding enough human milk or formula to correct it.[11])

After your baby is born and you are both deemed medically stable by your health professionals, SSC should be initiated. This means your towel-dried, naked baby is placed prone (belly down) on your bare chest, covered with a blanket and with their head turned to the side and slightly tipped up. Contact should last until the end of the first breastfeeding session.[12] While Baby Friendly USA and the WHO encourage doing SSC for a full hour or more, the original studies upon which this recommendation is based did not require a full hour, just to the end of the first breastfeeding session.[13] It's up to you how long you want to do SSC. You can do it later with your baby in a diaper. Partners and other family members can do SSC as well.

There is a very important caveat to SSC in that it can result in accidental infant falls from bed and rare cases of infant suffocation and death if the baby's breathing passage becomes obstructed, particularly if the parent falls asleep.[14] To practice safe SSC, the AAP recommends the following:[15]

1. A trained nurse should provide one-on-one supervision during the first two hours of SSC and breastfeeding to watch for signs of infant stress such as altered breathing patterns, activity, color, tone, and position.

2. Nurses should monitor mothers for signs of fatigue, illness, or inability to hold their infant.

3. Parents doing SSC should sit upright in a well-lit room to reduce their risk of falling asleep.

4. If the parent doing SSC needs to sleep, their baby should be placed in an empty bassinet, swaddled, flat on their back, while another alert support person is responsible for their care.

5. If the parent is alone and feels at risk of falling asleep with their baby, they should inform their nurse that they require nursery services so they can get a few hours of sleep to be more alert to safely care for their baby.

To read the full policy, scan the QR code.

Parent slightly reclined
while baby lies prone
on the chest

Head positioned to
one side and tilted up
toward you

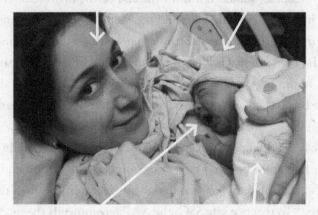

Nose and mouth
unobstructed

Baby covered with
blanket and snug hat
to keep warm

Safe Skin-to-Skin Positioning

Early Initiation of Breastfeeding Within the First Hour

After being placed skin to skin, your baby should be hungry and start root-ing to find your nipple. If mom and baby are medically stable, the first breastfeeding should occur within the first hour; this has been shown to promote sustained breastfeeding.[16] Babies are born with the reflex to crawl to the breast and latch on the nipple, called the "breast crawl," which can be seen in videos online.[17] Not all babies spontaneously do this, and it is not required for successful breastfeeding. You can support their body and head to crawl or simply place them close to your breast to latch.

Sometimes, maternal or newborn health concerns cause delays in this initial SSC and breastfeeding. If it does not happen immediately after birth, don't worry—your baby will still have the instinct to nurse and bond when you are together again.

Achieving Optimal Breastfeeding Position and Latch, and Ensuring Adequate Nursing Time

One of the most important factors in getting breastfeeding started well is a good latch, because it is helpful to both your enjoyment of nursing and your baby's ability to remove milk. A "good latch" may initially feel sensitive or tender but should not be painful; discomfort should not be more than 1 to 3 out of 10. Some babies latch easily and have a strong, effective suck; others need more assistance with latching from a lactation professional or trained nurse. If breastfeeding is ineffective and help is not available, or you're separated for more than two hours, you can manually express and collect your colostrum to feed to your baby.

HOW TO PROTECT MILK SUPPLY
IF LATCH IS INEFFECTIVE

If your baby is not latching well on either or both breasts:

1. Hand-express colostrum from each breast and feed it to your baby using a spoon, syringe, or bottle nipple. (Note: Hand-expressing both breasts stimulates milk production by removing milk from your body. Sometimes the expressed colostrum is not enough; if you are getting only drops of colostrum, you will need to supplement. Note that 5 mL or 1 teaspoon of colostrum contains 3 calories, while your baby's body is burning about 300 calories per day. Mature milk and formula contain 5–7 calories per teaspoon.)

2. Attempt direct breastfeeding at the next feed. If the latch is ineffective again, repeat step 1.

3. Seek latching assistance from a lactation professional.

4. If hand expressing is not desirable or effective, and your baby continues to not latch, fifteen minutes of pumping with a double electric pump at least six times a day, including once at night, has been shown to promote earlier onset of lactogenesis II and increased milk production.[18] We recommend pumping at least every three hours.

It is also important to choose a breastfeeding position that works for you and your baby; scan the QR code for good positioning options. Mothers who deliver vaginally may find the cross cradle or laid-back position most helpful for learning to latch; side lying is also a good option, if vaginal pain makes sitting difficult. Those who deliver by cesarean may find the football hold more comfortable, as it keeps pressure off their incision.

After birth, as we've discussed, your baby will likely enter a deep recovery sleep, which can last for eight to twelve hours. In some cases, babies remain very sleepy or uninterested in breastfeeding and need to be awakened every three hours to feed, in order to ensure adequate time nursing. Some babies are simply too tired to nurse effectively (see ways to wake up a sleepy newborn at the QR code below). Sometimes, however, sleepiness or lethargy are signs of low blood sugar.[19] If in doubt, your baby's blood sugar should be checked by a nurse. If a baby is sleepy because of low blood sugar, they will need to be supplemented with oral glucose, banked donor milk, and/or formula, or even IV glucose if it is severe.

To get breastfeeding off to the best start—and maximize the chances of successful breastfeeding—it is important to learn the basics of breastfeeding positioning, latching, and feeding on demand in response to your baby's hunger cues. You can find our guide by scanning the QR code on page 131.

HAND EXPRESSION FOR PROMOTING BREASTFEEDING

Hand expression of milk or pumping in addition to direct breast-feeding can promote sustained breastfeeding. One trial found that **fifteen minutes of hand expression or pumping done once at any**

time between twelve and thirty-six hours after delivery was associated with high breastfeeding rates.[20] Ninety-six percent of mothers who hand-expressed and 72.7 percent of those who pumped were still breastfeeding at two months.

HELPFUL MODIFICATIONS FOR CESAREAN AND COMPLICATED BIRTHS

Approximately 32 percent of US mothers and 21 percent of mothers worldwide deliver their babies surgically (by cesarean).[21] Mothers who deliver surgically or have complicated vaginal births (e.g., vacuum assistance, excessive blood loss, perineal tears, etc.) often need extra support. Most who deliver by cesarean are awake with epidural anesthesia, so those who are medically stable may have the option to do a modified version of SSC that keeps the baby away from the surgical incision, immediately after delivery, with assistance from a nurse. However, if you have to wait a few hours until you are ready, SSC will help breastfeeding just the same.[22]

Newborns born by cesarean or in very fast vaginal births tend to spit up more and may have transient problems with breathing due to amniotic fluid in the lungs and stomach that doesn't get squeezed out during delivery. This can make feeding challenging. Excess fluid can be suctioned with a bulb syringe from your baby's nose and mouth. Alert your health professionals if you are concerned about your baby's breathing or excessive spit-up.

Addressing Nipple Pain

Nipple pain occurs in 80 percent of breastfeeding mothers after delivery and is a common reason why women stop breastfeeding.[23] The most common causes are suboptimal positioning and latch, infant mouth anatomy (e.g., small mouth, tongue tie, high palate), flat or inverted nipples (see page 138), and strong infant suction.[24] Friction during feeds can lead to skin breakdown (abrasions), deep wounds (fissures), and infection. Getting early lactation professional help is crucial to preventing or minimizing nipple pain and trauma. Scan the QR code to learn more about nipple care.

CLUSTER FEEDING: WHAT IS NORMAL?

At some point, you may be told your baby is "cluster feeding." The Academy of Breastfeeding Medicine defines cluster feeding as "several short feeding sessions close together," usually lasting for a period of two to four hours a day. Normal cluster feeding may be important to increasing milk supply and meeting your infant's growing needs, as it signals your body to produce more milk.

What is normal cluster feeding?

- It happens *after* a mother's full milk supply is in.
- It is limited to about two to four hours a day, usually in the late afternoon or evening.
- Baby has the normal number of six to eight wet diapers and three or more dirty diapers a day.
- Baby is gaining weight appropriately.

However, not all frequent or prolonged feeding is cluster feeding. Constant breastfeeding all day long, especially for several days or weeks, may be a sign of inadequate feeding.[36] Newborns who are getting enough to eat are satisfied in between feeds during the day, fall off the nipple after a twenty-to-thirty-minute feeding, and sleep sixteen to eighteen hours a day in between feeds that fall every two to three hours.[25] Parents whose children became seriously underweight have written to us about their babies breastfeeding every one to two hours for thirty to sixty minutes each time, or continuously for hours. Often, a health professional told them this was normal cluster feeding. It wasn't until their babies were growing poorly, losing weight, obviously ill, or needing hospitalization that they were informed their babies did not get enough nutrition.

The ABM's supplementation guidelines state that an infant "who is fussy at night or constantly feeding for several hours" are situations where supplementation is "NOT INDICATED [their emphasis],"[26] with a brief mention of cluster feeding being "normal newborn behavior that should warrant a feeding evaluation to observe the infant's behavior at the breast and the comfort of the mother to ensure that the infant is latched deeply and effectively." The ABM provides no specific guidelines on checking weight, colostrum volumes, or blood tests to see if supplementation is needed when constant feeding for several hours occurs. Effective latching only improves milk transfer if there is milk there in the first place.

After several years of negative media coverage of breastfed infants developing serious complications when persistent hunger was dismissed by health professionals,[27] Baby-Friendly USA published a blog article in which the senior author of the ABM supplementation guidelines was quoted as saying that signs of persistent hunger in a breastfed newborn after the first day—even when weight loss or other clinical values are normal—*are* reasons to supplement.[28] If your baby is crying frequently or nonstop despite breastfeeding, or showing other HUNGRY signs (see page 151), your child may not be receiving adequate breast milk and likely needs supplementation.

THE IMPORTANCE OF ADEQUATE SLEEP
FOR SUCCESSFUL BREASTFEEDING

Self-care and getting adequate sleep are important not only for taking care of yourself and your baby but also for optimizing milk production and successful breastfeeding. Birthing parents often labor for more than twenty-four hours and are then required to take on full responsibility for their newborn's care immediately after birth, around the clock. Getting sleep in the hospital while you have assistance—especially if you have little support at home—will make you better able to go home and care for your baby. Getting adequate sleep once home also makes breastfeeding more sustainable; if your breastfeeding regimen is causing sleep deprivation that disrupts your well-being, you're unlikely to continue.

If you are suffering from severe sleep deprivation, we recommend getting a five-to-six-hour block of uninterrupted sleep, beginning right after a nursing session. Your support person will have to care for and feed your baby while you are sleeping with either pumped milk or formula, depending on your preference and what's available. While regular nursing is important for maintaining milk supply (see page 158), missing *one* feeding session to get sleep will not interfere with your milk production and may reduce stress, which has been associated with impaired milk production.[29] *So many* mothers have told us that getting this block of sleep saved their breastfeeding relationship, because profound sleep deprivation made them want to stop. This one five-hour sleep session can be scheduled into your daily routine for as many days as you want during a time that works best for you. See page 258 for more on how to manage milk supply around this block of sleep. Both sleep and milk removal are important for maintaining milk supply, and you will need to figure out how best to balance both.

FINDING YOUR OWN BREASTFEEDING
RHYTHM AND DEVELOPING A ROUTINE

Developing your own breastfeeding routine in response to your baby's hunger cues helps sustain milk production, ensures adequate feeding, and can eventually allow breastfeeding to seamlessly fit into your life. Following lactogenesis II, infants will consume more milk and should be satiated after most feeds. They will fall asleep after their full feeding and will sleep contentedly until their next feed in about two to three hours. Feed "on demand" or when they appear hungry, but at least every three hours. These feeding intervals can start to lengthen as they take larger volumes per feed.[30] Some babies will always eat about every 3 hours, though their feedings will become much shorter due to greater efficiency.

During the first two weeks, there will be some babies who are still very sleepy and need to be woken every three hours. Your pediatrician should examine your baby and their weight gain if they don't wake up to feed most of the time, in order to ensure they are getting enough milk to provide the energy to feed.

If you have an oversupply (meaning your milk supply is significantly more than what your baby needs), then your baby may only want to nurse on one side because they received enough milk from one breast. If your baby isn't willing to take the second breast, the feeding can end. Your other breast may be uncomfortably full; if the discomfort is severe, you can pump—but pump just enough to reduce the pressure. Completely emptying the breast can result in overproduction of milk, causing even more fullness and discomfort. For the next feeding, start on the side that was not fully drained.

For those with an oversupply who are trying to match their milk production with their baby's demand, leaving some milk behind will slow down milk production to the amount their baby requires. Alternatively, those working to increase their supply, pumping after nursing to "empty" can stimulate higher milk production.

Some parents take advantage of the first two weeks after lactogenesis II, when oversupply is more common, to build a freezer supply of milk; then they cut back on pumping once they have the reserve they need. But keep in mind that pumping after nursing can cause overproduction of milk that results in engorgement, milk stasis, and increased risk for breast infection called mastitis.[31] If you experience discomfort due to excessive breast fullness, you should reduce pumping.

BUILDING A FROZEN SUPPLY OF BREAST MILK

To build a freezer supply of milk without the risk of oversupply:

1. Pump for 10 minutes *immediately* after nursing at the first and second morning feedings, when milk quantity is highest.

2. If you are unable to pump immediately, wait until the next feeding and try again. Pumping any later may interfere with the amount of milk available at your baby's next feeding.

3. Collect and store the extra milk for freezing. The amount will be small, but within 4 to 7 days your supply should increase slowly, without oversupply. This can be continued as long as desired.

4. Once you are done building your freezer supply, gradually reduce your pumping regimen.

Sample Schedule for Building a Frozen Milk Supply

7 AM	10 AM	1 PM	4 PM	7 PM	10 PM	1 AM	4 AM
B + P for 10 minutes	B + P for 10 minutes	B	B	B	B	B	B

B = Breastfeed, P = Pump. You can be flexible with these times.

Feeding on demand does not mean you have no influence over your baby's feeding regimen. If your breasts are full and uncomfortable, it's fine to wake your baby to feed earlier.

Over time, your baby may begin sleeping longer at night (4–6 hours to start with) and taking larger feedings during the day. The amount of milk your breasts can store also influences how long you can go without removing milk and still maintain a full supply; this amount can vary.[32] It is essential to avoid prolonged engorgement because of feedback inhibitor of lactation, the hormone present in milk that can direct the breasts to decrease milk production.[33] For most people, this may require going no longer than three to four hours without removing milk during early lactation and no longer than five hours later on.

Babies do two types of sucking—nutritive and nonnutritive. Nutritive sucking means that the baby is drinking milk, and nonnutritive sucking is sucking with little milk transfer. Babies start out feeding by sucking quickly until the milk releases or lets down; then you may notice the nutritive feeding pattern—about one suck per second, followed by a pause during which the baby swallows (which sounds like a puff of air—"*kuh*"—accompanied by movement of the jaw and throat), and then a breath. This will repeat rhythmically until the flow of milk slows. Nonnutritive sucking patterns are about two or three sucks (or more) per second and may begin near the end of the feeding, when the baby is full and sucking for comfort.

Babies start a feeding looking hungry and then typically release the final breast, after twenty to thirty minutes, appearing satisfied. You can either wait for this to happen, or you can end the feeding by breaking the seal with a clean finger gently inserted between their mouth and your breast (just pulling the baby off can cause nipple trauma and pain). There are no hard and fast rules about nursing routines because every breast has different storage capacity and every baby has their own appetite and style of eating—some babies guzzle their meals, while others take their time. As long as your baby is growing well, and your routine is working for you, you're officially breastfeeding successfully!

Keep in mind that short (≤10 minutes total) or long (≥45 minutes) feedings are not typical at this stage. While they can happen occasionally, they may be signs of insufficient milk intake. Similarly, once your milk is in, babies that eat fewer than eight times a day or more than eleven times a day may not be consuming enough milk. In those cases, evaluation by a pediatrician and a lactation consultant with a weighted feed would be helpful; if necessary, a milk-increasing plan and supplementation can be implemented. Keep in mind that the amount you produce varies throughout the day; the lowest volumes typically occur in the late afternoon or early evening, and the highest in the early mornings.

Once your baby is getting their full milk requirement, diaper counts will better reflect adequate hydration and feeding. **Wet diapers indicate a baby's hydration status, and the number of dirty diapers indicates their nutritional status.** For the first six weeks or so, expect six to eight heavy wet diapers a day and at least three yellow, seedy stools a day, which change from day to day. There may be a few days when dirty diapers may be lower than normal even though a baby is still getting their full nutritional needs met. They will often catch up in the subsequent days.

GRAZERS

A few babies are what we call "grazers": babies who will breastfeed for ten to fifteen minutes, fall asleep quickly, and then wake up two hours later or sooner to feed again, around the clock. There is an important difference between a grazer and a baby who is not getting sufficient milk. Grazers are getting their full milk supply, appear happy and satisfied between feeds, and are growing appropriately.

There is nothing inherently wrong with this pattern, but it can be very tiring, and ultimately is unsustainable. We feel that if something isn't working for either member of the breastfeeding relationship, it's important to make a change. Work with an LC to improve this nursing pattern, as burnout is not helpful for long-term breastfeeding.

FOLLOWING YOUR BABY'S GROWTH OVER THE FIRST WEEKS TO MONTHS

Once a baby is receiving their full milk requirement, you may still wish to monitor their weight, especially if you have concerns about adequate feeding. For those with concerns about low milk supply, you can confirm weight gain by weighing them on a home scale. Simply weigh your baby naked every day at the same time for one week. Healthy weight gain is about 1 ounce a day (0.85–1.15 oz), or 6–8 ounces per week, until around four months when it slows slightly.[34]

Once you have confirmed that your baby is gaining about 6–8 ounces a week, you can reduce at-home weight checks. If you are still concerned about weight gain, you can weigh them once a week for four weeks. The Newborn Weight Loss Tool (or NEWT) website at www.newbornweight .org can also help you track weight gain over the first thirty days (see the tab at the top, next to the "First 3–4 days" tab). Although the NEWT is not tied to long-term outcomes, it is the best tool we have to approximate healthy newborn growth. According to the NEWT, newborn infants at the 50th percentile regain their birth weight by about a week and gain about 23 percent more than their birth weight by four weeks, or about 7 ounces per week for a 3.5 kg (7.7 lb) newborn. If your baby is at the 50th percentile of growth or above (green line in NEWT) and appears happy and satisfied with their feedings, your baby is likely receiving all the nutrition they need.

If your baby is gaining weight appropriately in their first month, monthly weight checks thereafter can confirm if your baby is following their growth curve. Your baby's doctor will weigh them at their one-, two-, six-, nine-, and twelve-month visits if your baby is growing well, and more frequently if growth is a concern. They will also plot the baby's weights on the CDC or WHO growth chart to ensure adequate growth for optimal brain development;[35] you can access these yourself at www.cdc.gov/growth charts/clinical_charts.htm. While some may cite the WHO growth chart as better than the CDC's with regard to tracking normal growth patterns of breastfed infants,[36] research has shown that the CDC growth chart outperforms the WHO growth chart when it comes to detecting poor growth associated with developmental problems.[37]

If your baby is gaining 5 ounces per week or less, their growth is slower than the 75th percentile line on the NEWT, or if your baby is showing signs of persistent hunger (feeding all day, for instance), even with apparently normal growth patterns on the NEWT, you can choose to supplement after nursing or wait and make an appointment with your pediatrician for evaluation. You can also get free weekly weight checks at many breastfeeding support meetings and pediatric clinics. Getting weekly weight checks can provide confidence to mothers who are unsure about adequate weight gain or low milk supply and help catch feeding problems earlier, increasing the chance of successfully boosting milk production.

LOW MILK SUPPLY AND HOW TO INCREASE IT

Problems with milk supply aren't only an issue before lactogenesis II. Chronic low milk supply after milk comes is common, and many report this as the reason why they stop breastfeeding. One study measuring the milk supply of mothers motivated to exclusively breastfeed with professional lactation support found two-thirds had low milk supply (arbitrarily defined as 440 mL/day for study purposes) in the first two weeks and one-third had low supply at four weeks, even with lactation support.[38] (For those who are curious, research shows that the average intake of exclusively breastfeeding infants is 788 mL every 24 hours, with a range of 478 to 1356 mL every 24 hours.[39]) Another study found that 15 percent of similar mothers had ongoing low milk supply at one month.[40] Forty to fifty percent of US mothers report "not producing enough milk" as the primary reason for weaning by six months.[41]

While some cases of low milk supply may be due to inadequate and/or infrequent breastfeeding or milk expression, there are also biological causes, some of which can be modified to improve milk supply.[42]

Non-Modifiable Risk Factors for Low Milk Supply

- More than thirty years old
- Prior breast surgery, especially reductions
- Insufficient glandular tissue
- Preterm birth
- Theca lutein cysts

- High BMI (modifiable only before delivery)
- Excessive blood loss from delivery (≥1,500 mL, but especially if ≥ 3,000 mL); while this can be corrected with blood transfusion, treatment does not necessarily improve milk production[43]

Treatable Risk Factors for Low Milk Supply

- High stress
- Hypertension
- Diabetes
- Hypothyroidism
- Polycystic ovarian syndrome (PCOS)
- Extreme malnutrition and dehydration
- Mastitis
- Estrogen-containing oral contraceptives (progesterone-only contraception does not interfere)
- Maternal medications, including some migraine medications, diphenhydramine (Benadryl), pseudoephedrine (Sudafed), phenylephrine, aripiprazole (Abilify), promethazine, methylergonovine (a postpartum hemorrhage drug), and corticosteroids (prednisone)
- Retained placenta
- Smoking, alcohol, and drug use
- Poor infant suck due to low tone, cleft lip/palate
- Poor infant suck due to tongue tie (see discussion below)

Helpful Tools

Steps that may improve chronic low milk supply include:

- Breastfeeding on each breast for ten to fifteen minutes or pumping for fifteen minutes about every three hours to maximally remove milk (see page 196).
- Power pumping one hour a day (see page 216).

- Not skipping the middle-of-the-night feeding, since milk production is usually highest at night.
- Addressing the treatable risk factors just mentioned:
  — Reducing stress, when possible, by practicing self-care and getting help with childcare.
  — Working with your obstetrician or physician to manage medical conditions associated with low milk supply, like hypertension, diabetes, PCOS, and hypothyroidism. Treating these causes may help low milk supply, although there are no trials available to tell us whether it will.
  — Avoiding estrogen-containing contraception and opting for progesterone-only options, like the Mirena IUD, Depo-Provera, or Nexplanon.
  — Avoiding tobacco, alcohol, and drug use.
  — Asking your obstetrician to check for retained placenta with an ultrasound. Spontaneous passage or surgical removal of retained placenta may improve milk supply.
  — Checking to see if any over-the-counter or prescribed medications you are taking harm milk supply on LactMed, the Drugs and Lactation Database, at www.ncbi.nlm.nih.gov/books/NBK501922.
  — If any of your medications interfere with milk production, consulting with your physician(s) to see if those medications can be switched to an alternative.
  — If your infant has persistent problems with latch even after consultation with an LC, having their doctor examine them for tongue tie, a condition where a small piece of tissue restricts tongue movement, as this can be surgically corrected. (Know, however, that according to the ABM, there is not enough high-quality research to determine whether surgically correcting tongue tie improves low milk supply or breastfeeding effectiveness and duration, although some data suggests it may reduce nipple pain for the mother.)[44]

— If your child has complex feeding problems like cleft palate or feeding aversion, working with a speech language pathologist trained in handling complex cases.

Unhelpful Tools

Many frequently suggested products to improve milk supply are backed by little scientific evidence supporting they provide any benefit. These include:

Herbal remedies. Many herbs have been used to try to increase milk supply, like fenugreek, milk thistle, moringa, and fennel seeds, to name a few. While these herbs typically aren't harmful, there is little scientific evidence showing them to be helpful.[45] If you plan to try any of these herbal supplementals and you are taking over-the-counter or prescribed medications, check with your doctor or pharmacist in case there are any important interactions.

Lactation cookies and teas. These are usually made with the above-mentioned clinically ineffective herbs.

Pharmaceuticals. There are medications that have been shown to increase prolactin levels, the hormone that promotes milk production, namely metoclopramide (Reglan) and domperidone (Motilium). However, evidence that these drugs are effective at increasing milk production is limited. According to the ABM, which currently does not recommend any specific medications to increase milk supply, high-quality evidence is lacking regarding these drugs, with available studies being small with poor methodology.[46] In addition, domperidone carries the rare risk of sudden death from a heart rhythm abnormality, especially in high doses; its use has been banned in the United States and restricted in Canada.[47] There have also been reports of severe psychological conditions from high dosages and rapid withdrawal from domperidone.[48]

TRANSITIONING FROM SUPPLEMENTED TO EXCLUSIVE BREASTFEEDING AFTER MILK COMES IN

Supplemental feeding is sometimes needed in the first week of life, whether for insufficient colostrum, a delay in milk coming in, or other reasons. But that doesn't mean supplemental feeding will continue to be needed. Many mothers are able to transition from supplemented breastfeeding to exclusive breastfeeding.

Once your milk has come in and your baby is effectively breastfeeding and appears satisfied with nursing alone, they are likely to decline supplemental milk. As long as they are having normal wet and dirty diapers, gaining weight appropriately, and appearing happy and satisfied most of the day, supplemental milk can be stopped and exclusive breastfeeding can resume.

However, some mothers will discover that even when their milk comes in, it may not seem enough to satisfy their infants (see "Low Milk Supply and How to Increase It" above). A slower increase in milk production is common and can often improve with good lactation management and additional pumping (see page 216).[49] If you are still having problems by day 7 after birth, see an IBCLC and your baby's doctor, as the first fourteen days of removing milk are critical for your supply.

WHEN EXTENDED COMBINATION FEEDING IS NEEDED

Some mothers find they are unable to achieve the milk supply required to exclusively breastfeed. While we encourage every parent who wants to exclusively breastfeed to seek out resources and work to increase their supply, it's important to think about whether your pumping and feeding regimen is working for you and your baby.

Mothers are often prescribed a triple-feeding regimen (breastfeeding, supplementing, and pumping every two to three hours) to increase milk supply, which is time intensive and causes sleep deprivation. Many who triple-feed experience a decline in their mental health, even progressing to postpartum depression or psychosis from the severe sleep deprivation. Furthermore, the regimen may not achieve the intended goal even after weeks to months of effort. If triple feeding is working, expect to see an increase in milk supply around day 4. We do not recommend triple feeding for longer than seven days, or for mothers who have risk factors for mental illness or have poor social support. Some mothers will not be able to cope with even a few days of triple feeding. If this is the case for you, you can reach out to a lactation consultant to see if your pumping plan can be adjusted. But it's also okay to stop if your mental or physical health is suffering. If you are not seeing an increase in milk supply in seven days, then you may have reached your ceiling for milk production for this baby. If your supply *is* increasing, work with your LC on next steps for maintaining this increased production. Scan the QR code to learn more.

While mothers can do many things to increase their supply, everyone's innate capacity to produce milk is different and can be limited by genetic and other biological factors that are out of their control.[50] If you find you are unhappy and spending more time with your pump than you are with your baby or family, ask yourself if what you are doing is actually best for you and your baby. Consider the fact that many mothers with partial milk supplies are able to happily breastfeed their babies for as long as they want while supplementing with formula. Some have even found that they were able to breastfeed longer with combination feeding than they did when they strived to exclusively breastfeed with a previous baby. Some use supplemental nursing systems to supplement at the breast; others use bottles; still others use both. Remember that as long as you are providing enough breast milk, formula, or both to meet your baby's needs, and you and your baby are *both* thriving from your feeding routine, then you have achieved what "best" infant feeding looks like for you and your baby. Read more about combination feeding in chapter nine.

Maya is my second low-supply nursling—not just low, dramatically low. I wasn't sure we'd make it this long and I'm thrilled to have made it over three years nursing this sweet baby! I just want moms struggling with low supply to know that your nursing relationship is more than the number of ounces you produce, and you can have a successful nursing relationship even producing very little milk.

—Joanna Kwaloff-Vedaa

MATERNAL MENTAL HEALTH: POSTPARTUM DEPRESSION AND ANXIETY

Shortly after birth, mothers experience changes in their hormones, and often their mood. The new demands of parenthood, sleep deprivation, and reduced time for self-care can cause sadness and anxiety often referred to as "the baby blues." At times, this can rapidly progress to postpartum depression and anxiety (PPD/A). PPD/A is considered the most common complication of childbirth, occurring in approximately 10–20 percent of postpartum women.[51] Suicide stemming from PPD/A accounts for 20 percent of maternal deaths.[52] In addition to harming the mother, PPD/A has known negative consequences for infant behavior, growth, and cognitive and emotional development[53] while also jeopardizing mother–baby bonding.

For mothers who prenatally intended to breastfeed, inability to reach their breastfeeding goal is a major risk factor for developing PPD/A.[54] When mothers are expected to cope with sleep deprivation, sore nipples, and a demanding breastfeeding schedule, all while recovering from the most intense physical event of their lives, it can cause things to snowball and turn early breastfeeding issues into bigger, more serious problems.

Many mothers who have sought support from our foundation have described being told that their infants will not be healthy or smart if they don't breastfeed. Some have been shamed by strangers, friends, family members, and even health professionals for using formula. They were told that they were lazy, that they would be giving their children substandard nutrition, and that if they simply tried harder, avoided formula, or got the "right education" from a lactation consultant, they would be able to exclusively breastfeed and give their child the "best." When these parents found that their breasts were unable to produce the milk their infants needed, especially if it resulted in feeding complications that threatened their infant's health, they experienced a *deep sense of worthlessness* and even suicidal thoughts.

If you are starting to experience frequent sadness or anxiety, get help and assess your situation. The Edinburgh Postnatal Depression Scale is a screening test that is available free to anyone at psychology-tools.com/test/epds. A score of 9 or higher, or any thoughts of suicide, require immediate medical/psychiatric care. For some parents, simple interventions like changing their breastfeeding schedule to get more sleep can be enough to improve their mental health. For more severe cases, antidepressant and anti-anxiety medications may be needed along with counseling.

If you are experiencing depression or anxiety because of not being able to exclusively breastfeed like you wanted, or because the regimen that has been prescribed to increase your supply is pushing you to your limits, or your feeding routine is keeping you from enjoying your new baby or your life, *then stop*. We are here to give you support, perspective, acceptance, and permission to stop what you are doing. You are *enough*. If your baby is thriving on a combination of formula and breast milk or formula alone, how you are feeding your baby is enough. Your worth as a parent is not measured in ounces, and your baby needs *you* more than they need your breast milk. You are the best kind of parent *because* your baby is fed what they need to thrive and because you've cared enough to sacrifice as much as you already have to give your baby the love and nourishment they need. Anyone who tells you differently is not looking out for you or your child's best interest. Find the people and health providers who think the same way and can give you the acceptance and support you need to find what "best" looks like for you and your family.

66

I always planned to breastfeed my babies. When I didn't make enough breast milk and my daughter had to be admitted to the NICU—jaundiced, dehydrated, and having lost 20 percent of her already tiny body weight—it was hard not to feel like it was my fault. I felt like I had harmed her by not trying hard enough and failing at breastfeeding. In reality, though, it was the intense pressure to breastfeed exclusively that did that. Not only did it make me put her at risk, but it placed me on a downward spiral of fear and shame when I couldn't achieve that goal, which, for me, was physically impossible . . . At the bottom of that spiral, I wanted to end my life. I got help, and eventually made the choice to switch to formula. I felt the pressure dissipate. Breastfeeding or not, I was enough . . . It was like being reborn as a new mom, without the crushing pressure to breastfeed. I realize that there's so much more—magnitudes more—to being a good parent than how you nourish your babies. And when it comes down to it, fed is best.

—Steph Montgomery

CHANGES IN THE BREASTFEEDING ROUTINE

Even when you have settled into a good breastfeeding routine, your milk supply is in, and breastfeeding is providing all that your baby needs to grow well, you might encounter a change in their usual feeding pattern. These changes are often normal and expected in breastfed babies.

Growth Spurts

One of these changes occurs during growth spurts, when your baby will be hungrier than usual in preparation for a brief period of more rapid weight gain. This can first occur between days 10 and 14. Your baby may want to nurse every 1.5 to 2 hours a few hours a day for a few days and then go back to their usual routine. This increased feeding frequency can stimulate the breast to increase milk production up to the maximum a mother is biologically able to produce, although the research on this is limited.

A growth spurt is different from cluster feeding in that this increased feeding frequency may last all day, rather than just two to three hours a day. You may worry that this increased frequency in feeding may be a sign of inadequate feeding. Remember, by this time, babies who are regularly getting their full milk requirement and growing appropriately will be in a fully fed state. This gives them a healthy caloric and fluid reserve to tolerate a milk supply that is slightly below their increasing nutritional requirements. Growth spurts are different for each baby, but expect them to occur around two weeks, six weeks, and at three months of age.

Breast Refusal

A more troublesome change in the breastfeeding routine is breast refusal. Feeding frequency can vary from day to day, particularly in the early days, but sometimes a baby will refuse the breast entirely, even though they are hungry. When this persists for multiple days, it's called a "nursing strike." There are theories for why this happens, but ultimately only the baby knows. Sometimes the taste of the milk changes temporarily during the menstrual period or if mastitis is developing. Sometimes colds can make breathing difficult during nursing; mouth infections like thrush can cause mouth pain during feeding; ear infections may make lying on one side painful. Some babies prefer looking outward during feedings, which they may find easier to do with a bottle.

Nursing strikes are usually temporary; babies can be gently coaxed back to the breast so long as they don't feel pressured to latch, which can prolong the breast refusal. *The most important thing here, for continued breastfeeding, is to keep your baby enjoying their time at the breast.* You can try:

- Offering the breast as a pacifier.
- Bottle-feeding skin to skin at the breast.
- Trying to latch when your baby is falling asleep or just waking up.

You can also take a break from offering the breast and feed expressed milk by bottle, then try the breast again a day or two later. If you are not able to fix the problem on your own, you may want to speak to a lactation consultant.

Ultimately it will be your baby's decision whether they comply with this plan, but you have a lot of influence, because most babies really enjoy nursing. We talk about this more in chapter ten, on page 265.

OTHER IMPORTANT MATTERS FOR ENSURING ADEQUATE FEEDING

Adequate feeding is not just about feeding your baby enough calories, protein, and fluids to support growth. It is also about providing their full requirements of vitamins and minerals and eventually introducing solid foods when they are ready, which are important for both infant health and brain development.

Vitamin D and Iron Supplementation in Breastfed Babies

The AAP recommends that infants who are born full term, exclusively breastfed, or combo-fed with half or more of their daily intake consisting of human milk receive iron supplementation by four months of age. It is also recommended that such babies be supplemented with vitamin D (400 IU/ day) within days of birth for healthy bone growth.[55] Both of these can be provided through infant vitamin drops or, after four to six months, fortified baby food when appropriate.

Iron supplementation is particularly important, as iron deficiency in the first two years of life can cause irreversible deficits in cognitive development that are measurable up to ten to twenty years after exposure to iron deficiency during infancy,[56] among other potential adverse effects.[57] A 2020 study found that among infants six to twelve months old, **54.3 percent had a calculated daily iron absorption below the recommended amount**, affecting 95.8 percent of exclusively breastfed, 72.2 percent of combination-fed, and 19.5 percent of exclusively formula-fed infants.[58] Breastfed preterm babies require iron supplementation from one to twelve months. Discuss your baby's needs with their doctor.

Introducing Solid Food

At some point, between four and six months, infants show signs of developmental readiness for solid food. Around this time, your baby's nutritional needs may exceed what can be provided by breast milk alone, and introducing solid foods alongside breastfeeding becomes necessary to support healthy infant growth and development. While the WHO and the AAP recommend introducing solid food at six months, this one-size-fits-all recommendation has resulted in infants developing poor growth when their parents complied, despite their infants needing more nutrition than breast milk could provide. Not all infants can wait for the six-month mark. The poor growth that results, also called failure to thrive, can impair cognitive development.[59]

Therefore, if your baby is showing signs of being developmentally ready, we recommend discussing solid food with their doctor. These signs include being able to sit upright with support, showing interest in and grasping for food, and having persistent signs of hunger despite breastfeeding as much as usual. If their weight percentile on the CDC or WHO growth curve is declining despite breastfeeding or combo-feeding as much as they want, this strongly indicates that they need solid foods to support their growth.

Meeting your baby's individual needs is more important than complying with the recommendation to introduce solid food exactly at six months. In fact, a systematic review of all the research on this matter has shown there are no differences in health outcomes between babies who are started on solid foods between four and six months and those started at six months.[60] Some parents have even been misled to think solid-food introduction at six months is optional, with catchy phrases like, "Food before one is just for fun." Food before one year is not just for fun. It is important for infant health and development.[61]

Infants typically are only hungry for and take in what they need for healthy growth. Just as for breastfeeding, feed solid food by following their hunger and satisfaction cues. While they may not eat a lot of solid food at first, giving them access to healthy sources of additional nutrition, like vegetables, fruits, whole grains, healthy fats, and lean meats, can prevent faltering growth when their nutritional needs exceed what breast milk and/ or formula can provide. It also sets them up for eating an increasing variety of foods important for their health later on. Introducing a healthy variety of foods usually results in a healthy growth pattern, which their doctor can confirm during well-baby checks.

Another reason to consider solid food before the six-month mark, if your baby is ready: for infants with a family history of food allergies and eczema, the AAP recommends introduction of baby-safe forms of allergenic foods like peanut products, eggs, and fish between four and six months to reduce the risk of developing food allergies.[62] Consult with your baby's doctor.

THERE ARE MANY ROADS TO SUCCESSFUL BREASTFEEDING

You may have a vision and maybe even a plan for how breastfeeding is going to go before your baby arrives. But just like everything else in parenting, what ends up happening may look completely different from what you imagined. Getting to know your baby and experiencing how breastfeeding fits into your family life can only start happening when your baby gets here. Your baby will be a unique individual with their own wants and needs. You will get to know them better than anyone and you should not be afraid to trust your instincts about what they need. Likewise, your breasts will be working in ways you have not experienced before, even if this isn't your first baby. It will take time to get to know how they work to support your baby's growth and how they will change over time as you go from birth to weaning.

It will likely take a few weeks (usually around four to six for first-time moms) to feel confident in your new breastfeeding routine. Once you get past the hard parts of learning this new skill and working through any issues, there is so much to enjoy about nursing your baby, and the first time they unlatch just to smile at you is something you will always remember. Enjoy the benefits, and you'll find it to be a special way to reconnect after work or any time you and your baby want to be close.

OTHER TOPICS FOR BREASTFEEDING FAMILIES

Information on the following and more can be found at the QR code:

- Early Latching Problems
- Tongue Tie
- Fast Letdown/Oversupply
- Plugged Ducts/Mastitis/Blebs
- More on Low Milk Supply and Slow or Low Weight Gain
- Milk Intolerance, Allergies, and Colic
- Nursing in Public
- Dysphoric Milk Ejection Reflex
- Weaning from Breastfeeding

they unlatch just to guzzle a couple more times before you fall asleep, relax a bit.

Enjoy the benefits, and you'll find it's best special with to reconnect after work or any time you need to pull them close.

OTHER TOPICS FOR BREASTFEEDING FAMILIES

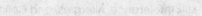

Information on the following may also be found at
bornfed.healthie.core.

- Why Latching Problems
- Tongue Tie
- Flat Nipples/Overactive
- Plugged Ducts/Mastitis
- Milk Allergies
- Supplements/Allergies to Foods
- Nursing in Public
- Oversupply with Breastfeeding
- Weaning from Breastfeeding

8

Pumped Milk Feeding

Pumping breast milk is essential for many lactating parents. About 85 percent of US mothers pump milk in the first four months of their child's life.[1] Some feed exclusively pumped (EP) human milk.* Others do so in combination with direct latching, where pumping takes the place of any missed feeds, or formula feeding. Those who EP generally pump as often as a baby feeds, with some variation, which we will discuss below.

Common reasons for pumping include:

- separation due to employment
- medically necessary separation
- baby not latching
- need or desire to monitor baby's milk intake
- pain or discomfort while breastfeeding

---

* If exclusive pumping is not your preferred way of feeding, but your baby won't latch, you don't have to resign yourself to pumping for the duration; some babies learn to latch weeks or even months later.

- to increase milk supply
- to relieve engorgement

The downsides of pumping, particularly exclusively, are that it can be time consuming and requires extra effort, such as washing additional equipment.

Pumping parents may receive warnings that feeding pumped milk through a bottle is "biologically inferior" to direct latching. For example, you may have heard about a popular 2015 hypothesis that a baby's saliva "backwash" while nursing can alter human milk's immune properties and

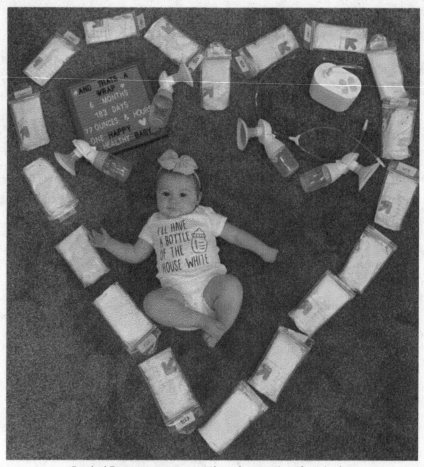

Rachel Boop commemorating six months of exclusive pumping for her daughter, Cecilia.

create specific antibodies for the baby. As of 2023, no research has demonstrated that retrograde backflow of saliva into the breasts directs the immune system to produce antibodies in breastfeeding human subjects.[2] Even if this hypothesis were confirmed, there are far easier ways for pathogens to enter a mother's body. Immunology research tells us that lactating mothers produce and secrete IgA antibodies in their milk when they are exposed to pathogens in the environment or via vaccination. These pathogens typically infect the mother through the respiratory and gastrointestinal tract. An infant with a respiratory infection may pass it on when the mother breathes in her child's respiratory droplets. An infant with a gastrointestinal infection can infect a mother if the pathogen from inadequately washed hands reaches her mouth. Both can result in maternal antibody production that does not require direct latching.

With regard to changes in nutritional content, while studies of breast milk show slight variations in nutritional content throughout the day and over the course of lactation, no research has shown any measurable health differences related to these variations.[3] So, you can feel perfectly safe feeding your properly stored milk pumped in the first month to, say, your now eight-month-old baby.

Other parents worry that bottle-feeding pumped milk may result in less bonding with their baby. Research shows that maternal–infant bonding is *not* determined by feeding type.[4] Bonding occurs whether babies are breast or bottle fed, or fed with human milk or formula, because it results from the countless acts of love that occur between parents and babies.

The take-home message here is that your milk is good for your baby whether it's from direct nursing or from a bottle. Freshly pumped milk offers similar nutrition and immune protection regardless of how it is given. While heating above 50°C (122°F), as is required for banked donor milk, might denature some of the immune proteins in breast milk, no differences in rates of infectious diseases have been demonstrated to result from feeding pumped milk.[5] So, if bottle-feeding pumped milk results in a thriving baby and parent, then you are officially doing it right. Don't let anyone tell you otherwise.

> "
>
> My exclusive pumping journey lasted six beautiful months. It was
> challenging, rewarding, and a huge learning experience for me
> and my daughter. I wouldn't change it for anything!
>
> —Rachel Boop

PREPARING FOR EXCLUSIVE OR PARTIAL PUMPING

If your goal is to EP, developing a full milk supply (typically about 25–35 oz/day of milk)[6] is possible through routine pumping of both breasts around the clock with at least eight pumping sessions daily. Remember, frequent and thorough milk removal signals your body to increase supply up to what is biologically possible for you at the time.[7]

The following is a checklist of things to learn and do to prepare for pumping. Our comprehensive guide to pumping is available at the QR code, where you can download and print this checklist and other helpful material.

Preparing-to-Pump Checklist

- ❏ Check which breast pumps your health insurance will cover.
- ❏ Research and purchase a breast pump that meets your needs.
- ❏ Measure your nipple at around 36 weeks to estimate your correct flange size.
- ❏ Purchase your estimated correct flange size and one size above it.
- ❏ Learn how to sanitize, assemble, and operate your pump before delivery.
- ❏ Learn how to express breast milk with your pump (but not before 37 weeks and only with clearance from your obstetric provider).
- ❏ Purchase desired accessories, such as a hands-free pumping bra.
- ❏ Set up your pumping station.

❑   Bring your sanitized pump to the health facility where you are
    delivering, in case you need to be separated from your baby or
    there is a question about colostrum/milk production.

CHOOSING A BREAST PUMP

Higher-quality pumps can be used on both breasts simultaneously, have
higher vacuum strength (between 220 and 350 mmHg, the maximum suction level), have adjustable suction and speed, and tend to be more comfortable. Many of these pumps have a "stimulation cycle" that mimics a baby's
pattern of rapid suckling that elicits milk letdown, then slows down and
increases suction strength to express milk, which can be helpful for some,
but not necessary for all.

Unfortunately, it is not usually possible to try different kinds of
pumps before buying, and some parents may be limited by cost or insurance coverage. Hospital-grade pumps are durable and powerful but are
the most expensive pumps available. Wall-socket-powered pumps are traditionally more powerful than battery-powered and manual pumps, but
some newer, wearable, rechargeable pumps now match their strength.
Wireless wearable pumps, however, have not been formally tested to confirm they work as well as plug-in pumps, and mothers have reported less
emptying of their breasts with wireless pumps.[8] Still, some find them
useful for getting additional pumping done while doing other things at
home and at work. Motors of non–hospital grade pumps also may wear
out with heavy use.

The first thing to consider in choosing a breast pump is your needs
as a pumping parent. If you have risk factors for delayed lactogenesis II or
you are returning to work after a brief maternity leave, having a portable,
high-quality, double electric pump will be essential for bringing your milk
in and pumping milk efficiently. A rented hospital-grade pump may be more
effective and reduce pumping time for those who need to pump more frequently, like EP parents who may need one until they wean. If you are an

experienced nursing mother with a history of ample supply and only need occasional pumping, you may get by with a manual pump. This chapter will outline the most effective ways to use a pump to maximize your supply. Scan the QR code to learn more about breast pumps.

PUMPING BREAST MILK WITH AN ELECTRIC PUMP

An electric breast pump is made up of (1) a flange, (2) a connector, (3) a valve membrane to prevent milk backflow, (4) a bottle or bag that collects the milk, (5) a motor, and (6) tubing. The *collection kit* refers to everything other than the motor and tubing. Some pumps also have filters that keep pathogens from entering the motor.

The most commonly used electric pump is the double electric pump. The following instructions apply to most popular brands, but always refer to the manufacturer's instructions.

1. Gather all the sanitized pump parts, bottle caps, and insulated freezer pack (if refrigeration is not immediately available).
2. Wash or sanitize your hands.

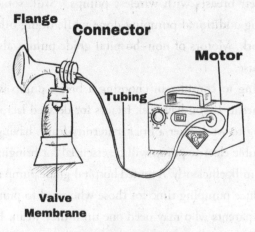

Parts of an electric breast pump

3. If your nipples are sore, lubricate them with a thin layer of nipple ointment.

4. Assemble your pump parts per manufacturer's instructions.

5. Place the flanges centered on your breast, making sure your nipples don't touch the walls.

6. If using a pumping bra, place the bra over the flanges and fasten it, making sure the suction feels as strong with the bra as without.

7. Attach the connector with the bottle or bag to your flanges (recheck your nipple placement before pumping).

8. Always turn the strength and speed dials to the lowest settings to begin pumping.

9. Turn up the strength of the suction slowly to the highest strength that is comfortable and removes milk efficiently, usually in the middle range (typically 98–270 mmHg).[9]

10. Some pumps have a stimulation sequence that starts automatically to elicit a letdown response. If your pump does not, you can mimic it if needed by turning the speed up to a high setting at the lowest vacuum strength.

11. Once letdown occurs, milk flow will increase. Pumps with the stimulation sequence will automatically switch to the stronger, slower pattern after two minutes. It's a good idea to switch to that pattern manually, once letdown occurs, for optimal milk removal.

12. Massaging your breasts gently with a free hand during pumping can help increase the yield from a pumping session. (A pumping bra frees up your hands to do this.)[10]

13. A pump should remove about 62 to 85 percent of the milk in your breast in fifteen minutes, the way the average baby would.[11] Once the flow of milk slows to infrequent drips, stop pumping. (Some mothers can initiate another letdown by continuing to pump for two more minutes, but if this doesn't happen for you, you can stop as soon as the drips become infrequent.)

14. Carefully remove the collection bottle or bag from the pump kit while avoiding contact with the milk.

15. Immediately cap the bottle or seal the bag and label it with the date.

16. Remove the collection kit from your breasts.

17. Store the bottle or bag in a freezer pack, refrigerator, or freezer (or feed by bottle) immediately.

18. Clean the flange, connector, and valve membrane with soap and hot water and store in a clean location to dry. Do not wash the tubing, as water can cause mold to grow. If there is condensation in the tubes, run the pump with the tubes connected and open to air for two minutes. Otherwise, replace the tubing.

19. Sanitize the flange, connector, and valve membrane daily using microwavable sanitizing bags, boiling, or a dishwasher on the hot water or sanitizing setting.

PROPER HUMAN MILK HANDLING, STORAGE, AND PREPARATION

We recommend following the CDC guidelines for storing and preparing human milk to keep your breast milk safe and uncontaminated.[12] *Cronobacter sakazakii* is a bacterium that occurs naturally in the environment. It can proliferate in powdered infant formula but has also been found in breast pump parts that have been inadequately sanitized.[13] *Cronobacter* can cause infections that are rare but often very serious—even fatal—for babies. In the United States, two to four reported cases of infant *Cronobacter* infections occur per year, but this is likely an underestimation given that reporting is not currently mandatory. *Cronobacter* in infants is set to be a nationally reportable disease in 2024.[14] Babies who are younger than three months, premature, and/or immunocompromised are especially vulnerable to this infection.[15] Human-milk-fed infants can develop rare *Cronobacter* infections from contaminated pump parts.[16] Scan the QR code for our complete guide.

PUMPING SCHEDULES

Milk production is stimulated by frequently and completely removing milk from the breasts. If you are exclusively pumping, we recommend pumping both breasts simultaneously for fifteen minutes at least eight times a day, about once every three hours, similar to a breastfeeding schedule. These pumping sessions do not have to be evenly spaced, but we do not recommend going longer than three to four hours without pumping until your milk supply is established and you learn how long it takes to become engorged. The goal is to pump well before you become engorged (indicated by uncomfortable breast fullness), as it can decrease milk production. If you are trying to increase your supply, do not go longer than every three hours in between pumping. One of your pumping sessions should be during a time when you have higher milk production. This is usually between 12 and 5 AM, when levels of prolactin, the hormone that promotes milk production, tend to be higher. For some, milk production is higher in the evening instead.

Sample Exclusive Pumping Schedule

7 AM	9 AM	12 PM	3 PM	6 PM	9 PM	12 AM	3 AM

Note the four-hour stretch of time between 3 and 7 AM, followed by a two-hour stretch between 7 and 9 AM. This allows for a slightly longer stretch of continuous sleep, followed by two pumping sessions two hours apart in the morning, when daytime milk production is highest.

If your milk supply is lower than you would like by day 7 postpartum, we recommend the following:

- Meet with an LC to get a full evaluation of your pumping plan and other risk factors that may affect your supply. Be sure to bring your breast pump to the consultation.
- Rent a hospital-grade pump until your supply has sufficiently increased.

- Incorporate one or two power-pumping sessions per day. (See below.)
- Decide how long you are willing to work on increasing your milk supply before making peace with the supply you have.

In general, if you do not see an increase in daily pumping volume after about seven days of committed effort, you may have reached your biological ceiling for milk production for this baby. While you can continue to follow this intensive pumping regimen, doing so for weeks without improvement can lead to severe sleep deprivation and mental health conditions.

Power Pumping for Increasing Milk Production

Power pumping (PP) stimulates milk production by draining the breasts multiple times during a one-hour period once a day, ideally when milk production is highest. It has been shown in a randomized clinical trial to increase milk volume when compared to an every-three-hour pumping regimen, almost doubling the volume per pump.[17]

Power pumping also provides pumping mothers a five-hour block of sleep each day (during which a partner feeds the baby expressed milk or formula in a bottle), something that is not possible with an every-three-hours pumping schedule. See more on this below.

For exclusive pumping moms, power pumping right after this five-hour block can make up for the missed pumping session during sleep. For parents both pumping and direct nursing, we suggest pumping for five to ten minutes to reduce engorgement (if needed), then nursing to completely drain the breasts. If power pumping right after waking is not convenient, doing it at any time will also be beneficial, though it will be most effective during high supply hours. Power pumping can also be divided into two thirty-minute sessions for those who have time constraints. If you are nursing directly, note that fully draining the breasts during power pumping may result in a smaller amount of milk being available to your baby at the next direct nursing session; make sure to offer them extra breast milk by bottle if they appear hungry.

Power Pumping for One Hour per Day After Waking

20 minutes pumping	10 minutes rest	10 minutes pumping	10 minutes rest	10 minutes pumping

Power Pumping for 30 Minutes Twice a Day During Highest Production Times

10 minutes pumping	10 minutes rest	10 minutes pumping

Below are two examples of a twenty-four-hour pumping schedule for EP parents who want to power pump. If you are directly nursing and pumping, you can substitute any pumping session with a breastfeeding session. Both of these schedules should be adjusted to what works well for you and your baby, but remember, power pumping when your supply is highest will give you the best results.

Power-Pumping Schedule for Exclusively Pumping with a Five-Hour Block of Sleep

7 AM	10 AM	1 PM	4 PM	7 PM	10 PM	10:30 PM– 3:30 AM	3:30 AM
Pump	Pump	Pump	Pump	Pump	Pump	SLEEP; partner feeds EM at 1:30 AM	1-hour PP

EM = expressed milk, PP = power pump

Power-Pumping Schedule for Nursing and Pumping Parents with a Five-Hour Block of Sleep

7 AM	10 AM	1 PM	4 PM	7 PM	10 PM	10:30 PM–3:30 AM	3:30 AM
Feed EM or BF then 1-hour PP	BF or P	BF	BF	BF	BF	SLEEP; partner feeds EM at 1:30 AM	Pump 5–10 min (if needed), then BF

BF = direct breastfeeding, PP = power pump, EM = expressed milk, P = pump

Power-Pumping Schedule for Exclusively Pumping with Two Mini–Power-Pumping Sessions

7 AM	10 AM	1 PM	4 PM	7 PM	10 PM	1 AM	4 AM
30-minute PP	30-minute PP	Pump	Pump	Pump	Pump	Pump	Pump

PP = power pump

Power-Pumping Schedule for Pumping and Nursing Parents with Two Mini–Power-Pumping Sessions

7 AM	10 AM	1 PM	4 PM	7 PM	10 PM	1 AM	4 AM
BF then 30-minute PP	BF then 30-minute PP	BF	BF	BF	BF	BF	BF

BF = direct breastfeeding, PP = power pump

Feeding Expressed Milk to Facilitate Sleep

Some nursing parents need an uninterrupted block of sleep to prevent exacerbations of a psychiatric or medical condition or to improve their quality of life. Having one's partner feed the baby expressed milk (EM) for one middle-of-the-night feeding allows the nursing parent a five-hour block of sleep that can ease sleep deprivation and stress. If there is no stock of frozen milk, then you may need to pump after nursing sessions during your highest producing times to have enough for this bottle, as shown below.

Feeding Expressed Milk to Facilitate a Five-Hour Block of Uninterrupted Sleep

7 AM	10 AM	1 PM	4 PM	7 PM	10 PM	10:30 PM–3:30 AM	3:30 AM	3:40 AM
BF + P	BF + P	BF	BF	BF	BF	SLEEP; partner feeds EM at 1:30 AM	P 10 min to reduce engorgement (if needed)	BF

BF = direct breastfeeding, EM = expressed milk, P = pump.

Expressed Milk Feeding During Work Hours, Pumping at Work, and Breastfeeding at Home

If you work away from home and breastfeed directly, you will need to pump while having your expressed milk fed by bottle during work hours. Ideally, you should start by pumping every three hours, and no more than every four hours. The goal is to prevent engorgement, as it can signal to your body to decrease milk production. Some parents can go longer, depending on their storage capacity.

Expressed Milk Feeding for Working Parents

7 AM	10 AM	1 PM	4 PM	7 PM*	10 PM	1 AM	4 AM	7 AM
BF	EM + P	EM + P	EM + P	BF	BF	BF	BF	BF

*Or upon arrival home. BF = direct breastfeeding, EM = expressed milk, P = pumping.

Do I Need to Pump in the Middle of the Night?

Middle-of-the-night (MOTN) pumping is important for most moms, who have their highest milk production at that time, especially for the first nine weeks.[18] Pumping at your highest producing time is your best opportunity to increase milk production.

If your supply is adequate and your baby is sleeping longer stretches, you may experiment with cutting out a MOTN session after nine weeks. You can do this gradually, by setting your pumping alarm increasingly later, or you can pump, go to sleep, and allow your baby or yourself to wake up naturally. If your milk supply is low or just enough, you will have to decide whether to prioritize sleep or milk supply, as delaying pumping can reduce milk production. If you are prone to plugged ducts or mastitis from breast engorgement, this spacing may be limited by the time it takes to become engorged.

Some mothers find that their milk production drops a few ounces if they eliminate the MOTN pumping; others don't. Unfortunately, it's not possible to predict how you will respond. You will need to experiment to figure out what works for you.

MANAGING MENTAL HEALTH AS A PUMPED-MILK-FEEDING PARENT

If your mental health is suffering because of your pumping regimen, we highly encourage you to adjust your plan. If lack of sleep is tipping you over the edge, drop a MOTN session and power-pump when you wake up. Ask your partner and family how they can further help with feeding and parenting tasks.

Some parents need to supplement with stored breast milk or formula in order to cut back on pumping for their mental health. Some find that their breastfeeding and pumping regimen is compromising their physical and mental health so much that they feel they must stop completely and only feed formula. Research supports that having an emotionally healthy mother is more important for you and your baby than maintaining a diet of exclusive or partial breast milk.[19] Know that you are doing what is best for your child by making sure you are healthy yourself. We support you. (Remember to use the online postpartum mood screening tool, the Edinburgh Postnatal Depression Scale, at perinatology.com/calculators/Edinburgh%20Depression%20Scale.htm.)

PUMPING ONCE MILK SUPPLY IS ESTABLISHED

As time passes, you may be able to pump less frequently while maintaining the same level of production.[20] Some can successfully sleep five hours once at night between pumping sessions, with a partner giving a bottle, if they pump or nurse enough to drain the breasts when they wake up. Others can sleep for six to eight hours straight without pumping and have no reduction in their supply, depending on their storage capacity. As you get to know your body, you can customize your schedule to do the minimum number of pumps while maintaining full milk production.

For some parents, it is easy to pump too often and develop an oversupply. Some mothers are happy to have this situation, as it means they can store extra milk for future use once they are done pumping. However, it's important to remember that overproduction may trigger inflammation, ductal narrowing (traditionally called "plugged ducts"), mastitis, and breast abscess.[21]

DROPS IN MILK PRODUCTION WHILE PUMPING

Drops in milk production are common for pumping parents, especially if the demands of life compete with time needed to pump. The following are some possible causes:

- Missed or shorter pumping sessions.
- Not getting adequate rest, calories, or fluids.

- Physical or emotional stress, such as going back to work.[22]
- Mastitis/breast infection.[23]
- Resumption of menses (usually temporary, lasting a few days).[24]
- Use of estrogen-containing birth control.
- Other medications (see chapter seven for a full list).

A drop in milk supply may also be the result of an issue with your pump. Remember to replace valve membranes and filter discs monthly because they wear out and cause suction strength to decrease. Pump motors, too, can wear out over time. Check your manufacturer's instructions.

If you experience a decline in your supply, you can power-pump for either one hour once a day or thirty minutes twice a day (see page 216). Alternatively, you can increase the frequency or length of your pumping sessions. Consult with your obstetrician, pediatrician, and an LC.

WEANING FROM PUMPING

When it comes time to wean from pumping, everyone's body responds differently. Some parents are prone to plugged ducts and must gradually wean to avoid them. Others can wean over a few days, with easy-to-manage engorgement that can be relieved with a few brief pumping sessions. While some parents must wean suddenly and unexpectedly for medical reasons, it's generally best to reduce supply and wean gradually. Make sure to care for your breasts during this process with cool compresses and over-the-counter pain relievers, if necessary. If you are experiencing pain, you may be weaning too quickly. Try giving your body a few days to adjust before further reducing your pumping regimen. Scan the QR code for detailed instructions on weaning from exclusively pumping.

In addition to physical discomfort, you may also experience feelings of sadness or grief around weaning from pumping. Post-weaning depression results from hormone changes in the body that occur when breastfeeding ends. Consult with your doctor if you are experiencing these symptoms.

9

Formula Feeding

According to a 2022 CDC report, 16.8 percent of families exclusively formula-feed from birth. By six months, 30.9 percent of babies receive both formula and human milk and 44.2 percent are fed formula exclusively.[1] Overall, about 83 percent of US families and 60 percent globally will use formula to nourish their babies within the first year of life.[2]

There are many important and valid reasons why parents choose to formula-feed their babies:[3]

Biological Conditions

- Prior breast surgery, mastectomy, reduction
- Taking medications incompatible with breastfeeding
- Inverted or flat nipples, or other variations
- Insufficient glandular tissue or low milk supply
- Inability to lactate

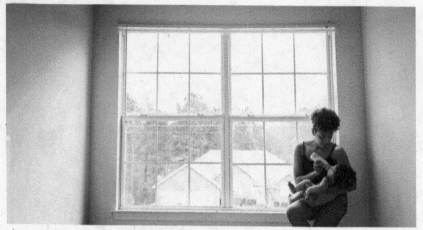

Kristen Umunna with her son Zakai

Psychological Barriers

- Mental health conditions
- Drug or alcohol addiction, active or in recovery
- Trauma related to breastfeeding-related feeding complications with a previous child
- History of sexual assault, abuse, or trauma
- Dysphoric milk ejection reflex, a condition that causes negative emotions with milk letdown

Social Factors

- Poor social support
- Poor workplace accommodations for pumping
- Wanting to share feeding responsibility equally between parents
- Desire for bodily autonomy
- The lactating parent's informed choice

Our goal is to provide a foundation of knowledge for formula-feeding families that helps them have a healthy and satisfying experience, while providing their babies the best possible outcomes. This chapter, along with chapter eleven on bottle feeding, covers information that parents do not readily receive on safe and optimal formula feeding, including:

- types of formula, including those with newer ingredients.
- how to choose a formula.
- how to reduce the cost of formula.
- how to safely handle and prepare formula.
- how much formula to feed your baby.

I planned on formula feeding . . . I support breastfeeding, but I won't do it myself . . . One of the most precious first memories I have of my daughter was watching her bundled up in the arms of her loving father; he cried tears of joy as he fed her her first bottle . . . We do things 50/50, even feeds. We slept in shifts and both of us, though still exhausted, were rested enough. Not everything was dumped on me like society had expected it to be. We were a team from the very start and that was important for us.

—Alix Dolstra

CHALLENGES FACED BY FORMULA-FEEDING FAMILIES

Despite the fact that most infants are formula fed at some point during infancy, research has shown that "33% of mothers felt guilty and 44% said they were made to feel guilty"[4] for formula-feeding. This highlights one of the many harmful effects of noninclusive public health messages like "breast is best," which creates a social hierarchy that labels breastfeeding the only moral option that "good" parents choose, thereby casting formula-feeding parents as less moral or less good.[5]

Another harmful effect is the lack of readily available noncommercial information about formula feeding. The *Washington Post* reports, "Many parents still struggle to find help once they make the decision to formula-feed. While breastfeeding parents have multiple resources available . . . formula-feeding parents often feel as if there is nowhere for them to turn."[6] Hospitals do not offer bottle- or formula-feeding classes. Parents often report that the only education they received is to "follow the directions on the can."

The reason formula-feeding resources are so limited is the 1990 Innocenti Declaration, which launched the global campaign to promote exclusive breastfeeding and called for a global ban on marketing of formula-feeding products, referred to as the International Code of Marketing of Breast-milk Substitutes.[7] Regardless of the ban's intent, the downstream effect is that it encourages health professionals to cast formula feeding as inherently risky, prevents them from providing formula-feeding education preemptively, and has created a societal bias against formula that leaves families that need it with few reliable sources of information. This scarcity of resources endangers the lives of infants and mothers whose health and well-being depend on its ready availability—and, ironically, leads parents to rely on formula companies for information.

I had more than enough support for breastfeeding, but very little support for switching to formula when I knew it was best for my own mental health, and for my son. I can't fathom telling a mom she'd better breastfeed or might as well be dead. But I was told this and I believed them.[8]

—Avery Furlong

"IS FORMULA SAFE?"

One of the concerns that families who have received the "breast is best" messaging often mention is whether formula is safe for their infants. Having accurate information on formula is particularly critical if their infant has developed a medical need for it but their educational resources have convinced them that formula is dangerous.

Formula milk is designed to be as close a substitute as possible to human milk and is the only acceptable alternative to human milk for babies. Infant formula is scientifically formulated to contain all the macronutrients (carbohydrates, protein, and fat), as well as essential vitamins and minerals, needed for healthy growth and development. Infant formula in the United States and many other countries has some of the most rigorous regulations of any product. In this country, the 1980 Infant Formula Act established requirements for infant formula nutritional content, quality control, labeling, shipping, storage, safety monitoring, recall procedures, and inspections in manufacturing.[9] Nutritional standards for infant formula are developed by the AAP Committee on Nutrition, and are then used by the FDA to develop regulations on formula manufacturing and sales. Internationally, infant formula standards are set by the Codex Alimentarius, overseen by the Food and Agriculture Organization of the United Nations, as well as the individual country's own guidelines.[10]

What all this means is that infant formulas go through years of extensive testing through randomized controlled trials to evaluate safety and efficacy in achieving healthy infant nutrition. Any new ingredients that are added also must be tested for safety. Once a formula is approved, every batch produced must meet a lengthy list of requirements.

However, while formula itself is safe, it must be manufactured, handled, and prepared correctly. Because of a voluntary recall of formula in response to several cases of fatal *Cronobacter* infections reported in formula-fed infants, and a subsequent shutdown of an Abbott Laboratories facility, there was a US shortage of infant formula starting in February 2022.[11] By that May, the nationwide formula out-of-stock rate reached 43 percent—in some states, exceeding 50 percent. Families reported having to drive hours to find formula, with some resorting to unsafe options like diluted or homemade formula.

Recognizing these limited options, the AAP and CDC condoned feeding unflavored, pasteurized whole cow's milk to standard formula-fed babies six to twelve months of age for up to a week with close doctor's supervision if they could not obtain formula.[12] Unfortunately, dangerous advice on substitutes nonetheless proliferated—and still does—on social media, parenting blogs, and websites. Such sources claim European formula bought through unregulated channels, unpasteurized milk from cows or goats, and homemade formula are safe or even superior to commercial infant formula. They are not.

In response to this phenomenon, Dr. Steven Abrams, Chair of the AAP Committee on Nutrition, wrote:

Pediatricians and the community should recognize that the use of infant formula is common but is not necessarily intuitive or without risks for misinformation . . . Websites and social media groups spread inappropriate advice related to unpasteurized milk, homemade formulas, and imported formulas with virtually no response from the medical or dietetic community. It is time that pediatricians and their allies such as registered dietitians take note that these sites are real threats to the health of many children, with an escalated effort at monitoring and respond as false information is propagated.[13]

Here are a few examples of unsafe practices that have gained attention on social media:

Using imported formulas sold by third-party sellers. European brands have become popular due to unsubstantiated claims that they are made with "higher-quality ingredients" that are "better for digestion" and "closer to breast milk."[14] During the 2022 formula shortage, foreign brands began to be safely imported to the US and are now available at most retailers. However, supplies purchased through third-party sellers on the internet are not regulated, and improper storage and international shipping may expose them to unsafe temperatures and conditions. Errors in preparation can occur if instructions are not printed in English or use different units of measurement.

Diluting formula to stretch it out. Almost half of US infants are served by the Special Supplemental Nutrition Program for Women, Infants, and Children (WIC), an important safety net that provides formula and food supplements to low-income families.[15] WIC, however, does not provide the full requirement of formula for exclusively formula-fed infants and even less to partially breastfed infants (e.g., 80 percent of the need in Texas on average), which can compromise infant nutrition.[16] Families most impacted by limited supply and rising costs of formula during the shortage reported stretching out their supply by diluting it with cow's milk or more water.[17] This can put infants at risk of malnutrition, electrolyte abnormalities, seizures, and death.

Homemade formula. Some parents make homemade formula from online recipes to save money; others do so because they mistakenly believe commercial formula is unsafe or substandard. Commercial formula manufacturers follow strict standards to match the nutritional content of human milk that are simply impossible for the average parent to replicate. Manufacturers also use special equipment for precise measurements and pasteurization.[18] Bacterial contamination is a major risk of homemade formula, especially when raw or unpasteurized animal milk is used.

Juices, sugary beverages, plant milks. Some families have given unsuitable beverages to relieve their infant's hunger, not realizing the risks. Not only can these fluids cause electrolyte abnormalities, but they can also result in protein and micronutrient deficiencies *because* they relieve hunger without fully meeting an infant's nutritional needs.

The FDA offers excellent evidence-based, noncommercially influenced information on formula, which can be found at www.fda.gov/food/people -risk-foodborne-illness/questions-answers-consumers-concerning-infant -formula.[19]

THE SIX MAIN TYPES OF FORMULA

Many new parents are not aware of the differences in formula types or even what type of formula to try first. Consumers can choose among six formula types:

Standard Cow's Milk–Based Formula

Most infant formula is made from cow's milk. It is what most infants are offered first, and is also the most economical.

Standard Goat's Milk–Based Formula

Infant formula made from goat's milk was approved by the FDA in 2023 and is now widely available at most retailers.[20]

Partially Hydrolyzed Formula

Labeled as "gentle" or "easier to digest," this formula contains cow's milk proteins that have been partially broken down into smaller proteins. This can help some babies who are unable to tolerate standard formula (indicated by excessive fussiness after feeds).

Hypoallergenic or Amino Acid Formula

These formulas have no intact proteins, only their amino acid components. They are intended for infants with cow's milk protein allergy, a hypersensitivity that can result in skin rashes or wheezing.[21] Hypoallergenic formulas have an off-putting taste and are the most expensive formulas available. Some insurance companies and WIC provide reimbursement for these formulas with a doctor's prescription.

Lactose-Free Formula

These formulas have the lactose from cow's milk removed and replaced with other approved carbohydrates.[22] Generally, babies do not have any difficulties digesting lactose. However, for babies with congenital lactase deficiency or galactosemia, rare inherited conditions that impair lactose digestion (the latter of which can result in buildup of toxic substances that injure the brain),[23] they require lactose-free formula to thrive.

Soy Formula

Made using soy proteins, these formulas can be used as alternatives to cow's milk formula for vegan and vegetarian families who prefer a plant-based option. Soy formula also can be considered for infants with cow's milk protein allergy, but 10–14 percent will also be allergic to soy protein.[24] Soy formula is also a safe alternative for infants with congenital lactase deficiency or galactosemia.

Note: Soy formula is not appropriate for premature infants as it does not contain enough calcium and other minerals to support their additional requirements for bone growth.

While this may seem like an overwhelming number of choices, you can be assured that most babies thrive on any of these options. The "best" one is the one your baby is doing well on.

PROTEIN AND CARBOHYDRATES IN INFANT FORMULA

Protein and carbohydrates are two of the main macronutrients in formula. Proteins are our body's building blocks and are required for countless bodily functions, and because the ratios of protein and carbohydrates in cow's milk are different than in human milk, cow's milk must be adjusted to match human milk. Protein in human milk consists of 80 percent whey and 20 percent casein, while cow's milk has the opposite ratio (80% casein, 20% whey). To support healthy growth, standard formulas are designed to match the whey–casein ratio of human milk.

Carbohydrates are a necessary source of energy for infants' rapidly growing brain, muscles, and organs.[25] Lactose is the only carbohydrate in human milk and the main carbohydrate in most infant formulas. Because there's a higher concentration of lactose in human milk than in cow's milk (7% vs. 4.5%–5%),[26] other carbohydrates like maltodextrin, brown rice syrup, corn syrup, corn syrup solids, tapioca starch, and sucrose must be added to cow's milk to match breast milk's carbohydrate content. Some European and American formulas contain only lactose, but it is not clear whether these offer any additional health benefits. Sometimes, carbohydrates are added because lactose must be eliminated, as in lactose-free formula. In the case of less palatable hydrolyzed formulas, other carbohydrates are added to improve the taste. Complex carbohydrates are also used in some formulas as thickeners to help with reflux.

Some parents have concerns about corn syrup, an approved added carbohydrate in some infant formula that is often confused with high fructose corn syrup, which is not approved for infant formula. At this time, there is little scientific evidence to inform us on whether these concerns have merit.[27] Corn syrup and corn syrup solids are considered safe by both the US FDA and the European Commission (EC).[28]

However you feel about the matter, you have many options regarding the type of carbohydrates that are in your infant's formula. Ultimately, what's essential for meeting an infant's nutritional needs is that the total carbohydrate content matches that of human milk.

For more details on other components of formula like fat and micronutrients, please scan the QR code.

Novel Formula Ingredients

You may also encounter marketing for formulas that include additional ingredients. Formulas with docosahexaenoic acid (DHA), arachidonic acid (ARA), prebiotics, probiotics, and bovine milk fat globule membranes (MFGM) are marketed as better at promoting infant visual and brain development than formulas without them. A2,[29] lactoferrin, and partially hydrolyzed whey (W-PHF) formulas[30] are marketed as easier to digest and closer to breast milk; W-PHF is also marketed as lowering the risk of eczema.

The FDA reviewed all the evidence behind each of these ingredients' claims and found the available data to be inconclusive.[31] Therefore, it does not currently require formula to include them. However, in May 2023, neo-natologists Erynn Bergner, MD, and Steven Abrams, MD, published an opinion calling for an independent review of newer data on DHA and ARA and to consider adding them to the list of required infant formula ingredients.[32] The European Union has required all formulas to contain DHA, but not ARA, since February 2020.[33] For a more detailed discussion of these ingredients, scan the QR code.

Ultimately, formula with novel ingredients is available, and which to purchase is your choice. However, if cost is an issue and buying a higher-cost formula that contains these ingredients compromises your ability to afford your baby's full nutritional requirement, it is better to buy a lower-cost formula and ensure healthy growth. There is far more robust data showing that simply meeting your child's full nutritional needs—through a sufficient amount of *any* FDA- or EC-regulated formula—is the essential ingredient for optimal infant health and brain development.[34]

HOW DO I CHOOSE AN INFANT FORMULA?

There is no single best infant formula. Most infants do well with standard cow's milk formula. If it's not tolerated, indicated by fussing after feeds, vomiting, or abnormal stools, then check with your baby's doctor. Often, hydrolyzed "sensitive" formula is tried next, then other formulas, if needed, per a doctor's recommendation.

The most important consideration in choosing formula is whether your baby is thriving on it. The next consideration is *the cost* and whether the family budget can accommodate it. The following table provides the relative costs, advantages, and disadvantages of different formula preparations.

Formula Product	Cost	Features
Ready-to-feed formula (2 oz single-serving or larger bottles)	$$$	• Liquid formula that **does not need *any* water added**. • Least likely to be contaminated given the sterilization process and minimal handling before feeding, especially if fed with sterile nipples. • Unopened bottles can be stored at room temperature. • Must be refrigerated and used within 48 hours after opening. • Must be fed within 1 hour of starting a feed. Any remaining must be discarded. • Recommended for infants < 3 months old and premature, medically vulnerable infants.
Liquid-concentrate formula	$$	• Liquid formula that **requires water to be added**. (Notice the bright red label.) Check manufacturer instructions. • If your tap water is safe, it can be used without boiling for healthy infants > 3 months old. • If you have doubts about water quality or a medically vulnerable infant, boil the water before mixing, then cool before feeding, or use bottled water. (See detailed instructions on page 236.)
Powdered formula	$	• Powdered mixture in a tub or can. • Must be prepared with a safe water source according to manufacturer instructions. • Can be prepared for individual feedings or a full day's worth if refrigerated and used within 24 hours. • Must be fed within 2 hours of preparation if unrefrigerated and within 1 hour of starting a feed; any remaining must be discarded. • Shelf life is 30 days after opening the container.

REDUCING THE COST OF FORMULA

Formula is expensive. In some parts of the world, even for those who need it, the cost of formula makes it an unsustainable option. It is important to note that *all* infant formulas sold in the United States and many parts of the world are required to meet strict standards to safely fulfill an infant's nutritional requirements. Therefore, whether your formula is brand name or store brand, organic, contains special ingredients, or doesn't, your baby is likely going to have the same health outcomes.

Why does the price vary so widely between brand-name and store-brand formula? It primarily comes down to marketing costs of brand-name formula being passed on to the consumer. Some of the cost is related to research and development, which includes research on novel ingredients—some of which may not yet have strong enough evidence supporting that they provide any additional benefits.[35]

The following are estimates of the average annual costs of infant formula as of December 2023:

Estimated Annual Cost of Infant Formula*

Type of Standard Powdered Cow's Milk Formula	Annual Cost
Name-brand ($1.42/oz of powdered formula)	$2952
Store-brand ($0.99/oz of powdered formula)	$1776
Out-of-pocket cost of name-brand formula for WIC recipients**	$590
Out-of-pocket cost of store-brand formula for WIC recipients**	$355

*Calculated from the estimated daily requirement of exclusively formula-fed infants (on page 244) plus 20 percent, to account for waste that occurs in real life. Actual costs will vary depending on formula brand and current market prices.

**Out-of-pocket costs presume the purchase of the 20% of an infant's full formula requirement not covered by the WIC program (although WIC does not typically subsidize store-brand formula).

Fortunately, there are a few ways to reduce the cost of infant formula:

- **Choose a store-brand formula.** They are less expensive than name-brand, organic, or non-GMO formulas and provide equivalent health outcomes. Even if your baby has been getting name-brand formula thus far, you can easily switch to an equivalent store brand.
- **Choose a powdered formula.** It is the most economical form of formula, followed by liquid concentrate, then ready-to-feed.
- **Buy in bulk.** Larger packages usually cost less per ounce. Some vendors offer discounts for monthly subscriptions.
- **Take advantage of coupons and free samples.** Contact the manufacturer to see if they have discount coupons or free samples.

PROPER PREPARATION OF POWDERED OR LIQUID-CONCENTRATE INFANT FORMULA

Proper formula preparation is *extremely* important. Adding too much water dilutes essential nutrients that affect a child's growth, health, and development. Adding too little water can result in gastrointestinal problems and constipation. Both can cause serious electrolyte abnormalities, seizures, and other life-threatening conditions. Inadequate sterilization of nipples, bottles, and formula preparation equipment; preparing formula with contaminated water; or poor handwashing before formula preparation can also lead to gastrointestinal infections.

Read the following guide as well as the instructions on your formula container. If the advice between the two conflicts, always follow the container's instructions. Always check the expiration date before purchasing or using the formula. Contact the manufacturer and/or consult with your pediatrician regarding any questions about preparation and feeding.

1. Determine whether your water is safe.[36]

Families living in the United States are likely to have tap water that is safe for formula preparation, as the country's public drinking water is among the safest in the world. You can confirm your area's water quality by calling the EPA's Safe Drinking Water Hotline (1-800-426-4791). For households that rely on private wells, the EPA recommends either getting the water tested or using bottled water.

Public drinking water generally contains fluoride to protect against tooth decay. However, most formula also contains fluoride. According to the CDC, feeding infants with formula prepared with fluoridated tap water may increase the risk of dental fluorosis (faint white markings on permanent teeth; not a health hazard).[37] Municipal and well water can be checked for fluoride levels to see if they are appropriate. If you are worried about fluorosis, you can choose low-fluoride bottled water, which will be labeled as deionized, purified, demineralized, distilled, or nursery water.

2. Sanitize the formula prep area.

First, clean and sanitize the formula prep area with a disinfectant. Wash hands with warm water and soap for twenty seconds. Place all your sterilized bottle-feeding supplies on the prep area next to your formula container.

Before first use, wash and dry the outside of the formula container, as dirt and bacteria on the lid can contaminate the formula once opened. Without touching the formula, visually inspect it for color, texture, clumping, or foreign particles; if you notice something unusual, do not use it, and report it to the manufacturer. (Make sure you're signed up for formula recall alerts as well.)

3. Boil your water (if needed).[38]

This may be one of the most confusing topics for parents. If your water is safe, what is the purpose of boiling it?

It is actually not about making the *water* safe—it's about killing pathogens that may be in the *powder* once the container is opened and used. Per
FDA regulations, formula powder is always tested for bacterial contamination before distribution. But it can become contaminated at home from
unclean hands that touch the formula scoop, from unclean surfaces during
preparation, or if used after the expiration date.

Boiling the water is particularly important to kill any *Cronobacter* in
the powdered formula. Because it causes rare fatal infections, especially in
babies who are less than three months old, premature, and/or immunocompromised,[39] the CDC recommends feeding such infants with ready-to-feed
formula. If this is not possible, preparing powdered formula in the manner
described below can reduce the risk of this infection. For healthy infants
older than three months, unheated tap or bottled water can be used to prepare formula while following the remaining steps.

To boil water:

1. Measure slightly more water than the amount needed into a pot.
2. Bring the water to a full boil.
3. Remove the pot from the stove and let water cool for about thirty
   minutes to **no less** than 70°C/158°F using a kitchen thermome-
   ter. (Mixing the formula at this temperature will kill any potential
   pathogens in the powder while maintaining the complete nutritional value of the formula.)

We recommend boiling enough water to prepare a twenty-four-hour
batch of formula. Making your formula in batches can save time and effort,
make mixing easier, reduce air bubbles, and reduce the risk of burns that
can happen when formula is prepared with hot water for each feed.[40]

4. Mix formula with water.

TO PREPARE POWDERED FORMULA

1. Pour the appropriate amount of (hot—**no less** than 70°C/158°F) water into your bottle (for single-bottle preparation) or pitcher or jar (for large-batch preparation).

2. Add the appropriate number of scoops of formula to the hot water. This is typically one loosely packed level scoop of powder for every 2 ounces of water (only a few special formulas recommend packing; check your container).[41] To remove excess formula, slide the scoop against the straight edge of the formula container or slide a clean knife across the top of the scoop. Be careful to not lose count while dispensing the scoops into larger containers, as errors can lead to under- or overdilution. Counting aloud may reduce errors. **If you have any doubt that you have mixed the wrong number of scoops of formula during preparation, discard it and start again.**

3. Mix the water and formula together thoroughly. After mixing, you will have more formula in the container than the volume of water you started with.

Your baby's formula intake is based on the total volume after mixing water with formula, which will be slightly greater than the fluid used to prepare it. But note: Research has shown that the volume markers on some infant bottles may be inaccurate, so it is important to confirm that your bottles are correctly marked by filling them with the correct volume of water measured with a measuring cup.[42]

TO PREPARE LIQUID-CONCENTRATE FORMULA

Mix liquid-concentrate formula with an equal volume of boiled water cooled to 70°C/158°F. As a reminder: For healthy infants older than three months, safe, unheated water is okay to use.

5. Feed your baby.

If you are feeding your baby immediately, pour the desired amount of formula into a bottle, cap it, and cool it under cold running water to body temperature—about 98°F/37°C. Check the temperature by squeezing a drop onto the inside of your wrist before giving it to your baby.

6. Refrigerate excess prepared formula immediately.

Place any *excess* prepared formula in the refrigerator right away; do not leave it out to cool before storing. It must remain refrigerated until use, preferably not on the door shelves where the temperature may be warmer. Use a refrigerator temperature gauge to ensure the fridge temperature remains between 35°F and 40°F (1.6°C–4.4°C). Note: Unused prepared formula must be used within twenty-four hours.[43]

7. Properly store your unused formula.

Once you are done with the powdered formula, place the scoop back into the container. Many containers have a scoop holder on the lid, to reduce the risk of bacterial contamination from the scoop handle once it has been touched. If there is no scoop holder, simply put the scoop on top of the powder with the handle up above the powder. Close the lid and store in a cool, dry place, away from direct sunlight.

Any opened but unused bottles of liquid-concentrate formula require refrigeration immediately and must be used within forty-eight hours.

Scan the QR code for:

- A printable checklist for powdered formula preparation.
- A printable guide to single- or multiple-bottle powdered formula preparation (after 3 months) without boiling water.

> ## HEATING COLD INFANT FORMULA
>
> Many infants don't mind cold formula. But if you choose to heat your baby's formula, warm it to body temperature by placing the capped bottle under warm water. There are commercial bottle warmers available as well, but check for recalls before using them. Avoid using a microwave to warm bottles, however; this can cause "hot spots" that may burn your baby's mouth.

FORMULA-FEEDING YOUR BABY AT BIRTH

Hospitals use sterile formula bottles and nipples, using new ones of each for each feeding. Each bottle holds 60–80 mL of formula. After your baby is born, skin-to-skin time can help stabilize their temperature and blood sugar levels. As your baby begins to show hunger cues, feeding them formula will help stabilize their blood sugar levels, too, and bottle feeding provides another bonding opportunity.

HOW MUCH FORMULA TO FEED YOUR BABY

There are many myths surrounding how differently breastfed and formula-fed babies feed. But all babies require the same nutrition and fluid volumes, regardless of whether they're receiving formula or human milk. Many parents have been taught that it is easy to overfeed with formula, but it is no more or less likely than overfeeding with bottled human milk—meaning not very, if you follow your baby's fullness cues and let them decide when they're done.

Day 1 (During Their Recovery Period)

Most newborns experience an eight-to-twelve-hour period of recovery shortly after birth where they eat less than their full caloric requirement.

Therefore, most babies lose a small amount of weight during the first few days of life. The average formula-fed infant loses a maximum of 3–4 percent of their birth weight; rarely, they lose more than 7–8 percent, with only 0.1 percent losing more than 10 percent.[44] Losing too much weight (>7 percent) puts newborns at risk of feeding complications, like excessive jaundice and dehydration,[45] which is why it's important to know how much formula to feed. An average-size newborn (7 lb) may take around **0.5–1 ounce (15–30 mL) every two to three hours** on the first day of life. Remember that their stomach is around 20–30 mL at birth but empties and slows digestion in response to hormones that signal hunger and satisfaction, respectively.[46] Some larger infants (8–10 lb), or smaller infants born with limited caloric reserves, may be hungrier for more.

If your baby is full term, follow their hunger cues and feed them on demand. (If they are preterm, consult with their doctor.) You can offer half an ounce (15 mL) at a time, pausing to check for hunger cues to know whether to offer more. Stop when your baby shows signs of satisfaction (see page 281). Their intake volume can vary between feeds, and the interval between feeds can vary slightly. However, in the first days, you should not go longer than three hours without offering a feed, even if you have to wake your baby up. The CDC recommends 1 to 2 ounces of formula for EFF babies every two to three hours in the first days, more if they are showing signs of hunger.[47]

Spitting up is common for all infants during the first days of life, as they are getting rid of any extra fluid in the lungs and the stomach. Spit-up contains a mixture of amniotic fluid, mucus, or formula, and it is not necessarily a sign of overfeeding. More accurate signs of overfeeding include milk running out of the mouth and spitting out the nipple (see page 283), which should trigger you to stop feeding.

Day 1 to 2 (After Their Recovery Period) to One Month of Age

Newborns know what they are hungry for. Once they awaken from their recovery period on day 1 or 2, they will likely be hungry for their full milk requirement, which for an average-sized infant is **2–2.5 ounces (60–75 mL) every three hours.**[48]

You can calculate your own infant's daily milk requirement by scanning this QR code.

Recommended Schedule of Volumes for Healthy, Term, Exclusively Formula-Fed Newborns[49]

Day 1	• Small to average-sized infants may take 15–30 mL (0.5–1 oz) per feed. • Larger infants or infants with limited caloric reserves may be hungrier; offer 15 mL (0.5 oz) at a time with a pause between to see if they are still hungry, as indicated by continued rooting or fussing. • Feeds should be given on demand, but go no longer than 3 hours without offering a feed. • Stop the feeding if an infant shows signs of satisfaction.
Day 2	• Average-sized infants may take 30–45 mL (1–1.5 oz) per feed. • Larger infants may take 45–75 mL (1.5–2.5 oz) per feed. • Smaller infants may take 15–30 mL (0.5–1 oz) per feed. • Feed on demand, at least every 3 hours.
Day 3 to 2 weeks	• Most infants will take 1–2 ounces per feed. • They will occasionally go 4 hours between feeds.
2 to 4 weeks	• Most infants will take 2–3 ounces per feed.

Remember to consult with your doctor regarding your baby's individual needs.

One Month of Age to When Solid Foods Are Introduced

After the first month, the amount of formula required increases by 1 ounce (30 mL) per feed every month, until the baby reaches a maximum of about 7–8 ounces (210–240 mL) per bottle feed and 32 ounces (960 mL) of formula in twenty-four hours.[50] See the chart on page 244.

If your baby seems to want more or less than this, you can discuss it with your pediatrician, who will monitor your baby's growth at every visit. You can also monitor your baby's growth against the CDC growth chart with a home baby scale. (We recommend the CDC growth chart as it outperforms the WHO for detecting developmental problems; scan the QR code to learn more.) Once your baby starts showing signs of hunger despite full formula feeding, they may be ready for solid food.

Daily Calorie Requirement by Age and Corresponding Formula Volumes[51]

Average Amount and Schedule of Formula Feedings in the First Year of Life				
Age	Average Daily Calorie Requirement (kcal/kg/day)*	Average Weight (kg)**	Estimated Daily Formula Requirement (in oz)***	Average Volume per Feed (in oz) and Frequency
0–1 month	110	4.47	24.6	2–3 oz every 3 hours
1–2 months	103	5.32	27.4	3–4 oz every 3–4 hours
2–3 months	95	6.05	28.7	3–6 oz 5–8 times per day
3–4 months	83	6.68	27.7	3–6 oz 5–8 times per day
4–5 months	82	7.20	29.5	4–6 oz 4–6 times per day ± solids****
5–6 months	82	7.64	31.3	4–6 oz 4–6 times per day ± solids

Average Amount and Schedule of Formula Feedings in the First Year of Life				
Age	Average Daily Calorie Requirement (kcal/kg/day)*	Average Weight (kg)**	Estimated Daily Formula Requirement (in oz)***	Average Volume per Feed (in oz) and Frequency
6–7 months	80	8	32 + solids	6–8 oz 3–5 times per day + solids
7–8 months	80	8.32	32 + solids	6–8 oz 3–5 times per day + solids
8–9 months	80	8.6	32 + solids	7–8 oz 3–4 times per day + solids
9–10 months	80	8.84	32 + solids	7–8 oz 3–4 times per day + solids
10–11 months	80	9.075	32 + solids	7–8 oz 3–4 times per day + solids
11–12 months	80	9.31	32 + solids	7–8 oz 3–4 times per day + solids

* The calorie requirements are averages between girls and boys; boys typically have higher caloric requirements than girls.

** The average weights are used to calculate the estimated daily formula requirement. For more accurate estimates, find the caloric requirement for their age, then multiply that by your child's weight in kg. Then divide this number by 20 kcal/oz to get the total daily formula requirement in ounces.

***Assumes 20 kcal/oz formula.

****Some infants may benefit from introduction of solid food between 4 and 6 months depending on their nutritional needs and to reduce the risk of food allergies (e.g., to peanuts, eggs, etc.). Consult with your baby's doctor.

REDUCING ALLEGED RISKS OF HEALTH PROBLEMS ASSOCIATED WITH FORMULA FEEDING

We discussed in chapter three how many of the advantages associated with breastfeeding are heavily affected by parental socioeconomic status, education levels, and child-rearing behavior. While it is true that when populations of babies are studied, breastfed babies on average do better than formula-fed babies,[52] in settings with access to formula, when breastfed and bottle-fed siblings are compared, the differences disappear.[53] This suggests that the improved health outcomes in breastfed children are likely due to their home environment and the child-rearing choices their parents make.

However, we know that this may not eliminate the concern that some parents have about the increased risk of various conditions that have been associated with formula feeding. Therefore, we have provided the following evidence-based guide on parenting choices that might reduce the risk of these conditions without breastfeeding, in order to offer options for parents who may feel anxious about these risks. It is by no means a validation of the inaccurate message that formula *causes* these conditions.

Ways Other Than Breastfeeding to Reduce Risk of Health Problems

Health Condition	Alternative Ways to Reduce Risk
Ear infections	• Using an upright position while feeding (see chapter eleven, page 279)[54] • Delaying daycare attendance until 24 months (when ear infections become less common)[55] • Treating GERD, if present[56]
Respiratory infections[57]	• Using an upright position while feeding[58] • Delaying daycare attendance (same as for ear infections)[59] • Completing childhood immunizations

Health Condition	Alternative Ways to Reduce Risk
Gastrointestinal infections	• Ensuring proper formula preparation, handling, and storage • Performing good hand hygiene and proper cleaning of feeding equipment during food preparation • Completing childhood immunizations
Asthma/reactive airway disease	• Using an upright position while feeding • Eliminating household tobacco smoke and mold[60] • Reducing maternal prenatal stress[61] • Avoiding newborn hyperbilirubinemia with adequate feeding[62] • Exposing children to household pets[63]
Childhood eczema	• Avoiding vitamin D deficiency[64] • Avoiding newborn hyperbilirubinemia[65] • Exposing children to pets and farm animals[66]
Child food allergies	• Introducing allergenic foods between 4 and 6 months[67]

Overweight/ obesity Hypertension Diabetes	• Responsive feeding (see page 281)[68]
	• After introducing solid food:
	  – Avoiding sugary and high-calorie foods and beverages
	  – Encouraging healthy diet and exercise

Intelligence/ cognitive development	• Fostering healthy brain development through safe and sufficient feeding • Fostering close infant–parent relationship • Providing educational enrichment
Cancer	• Avoiding needless exposure to ionizing radiation (X-rays and CT scans) and carcinogens (e.g., pesticides, benzene, paint thinner, paints, tobacco products), during pregnancy and after birth[69] • Avoiding alcohol, cannabis/marijuana products, and illicit drug use during pregnancy[70] • Avoiding newborn hyperbilirubinemia[71]
SIDS	• Using pacifiers[72] • Ensuring safe sleep practices[73] (no bed sharing; child sleeps alone, on their back, in a crib)

HANDLING FORMULA SHAMING

One of this book's missions is to change public attitudes about infant feeding and to increase awareness of the wide diversity of biology and circumstances that affect how parents ultimately "best" feed their babies. Unfortunately, public perceptions that breastfeeding versus formula feeding is simply a matter of choice, education, or effort have caused those who formula-feed to be judged and shamed. Often, formula feeding is not a choice. As one mom, Kristen Umunna, put it:

> I put her to the breast on demand at home as I was told in my Baby-Friendly hospital. Yet, she kept crying and crying . . . When the pediatrician walked in the room at our clinic visit . . . she told us we had to take her to the hospital immediately . . . She was diagnosed with jaundice, hypernatremia, hypoglycemia, and dehydration. She was critically ill because I was not making any breast milk . . . I've never felt so worthless in my mothering journey . . . I was eventually diagnosed with [postpartum depression] and was advised by my doctor to switch to all formula milk . . . I did so and the heavy depression began to lift. Formula feeding was the best decision for me and my mental health. We were both thriving for the first time, and it was glorious.

The best way to combat shaming and bullying is to reject the validity of the message that formula feeding is harmful or inferior and expose its fallacies. The next best way is to teach as many people as possible a more positive and inclusive perspective that reminds them of the most important goal of infant feeding. According to the AAP, "The child's nutrition in the first 2 years of life are crucial factors in a child's neurodevelopment and lifelong mental health. Child and adult health risks, including obesity, hypertension, and diabetes, may be programmed by nutritional status during this period . . . The failure to provide adequate macronutrients or key micronutrients at critical periods in brain development can have lifelong effects on a child."[74] In other words, according to child nutrition experts, "fed is best." Safely and fully fed infants have the highest potential for having the best immunological, behavioral, psychological, cognitive, and overall health outcomes. If achieving this goal requires you to use formula, or if you simply choose formula, it still means you, in fact, *are* giving your child the best.

Know that if you use formula at some point, you are part of the majority of parents on this planet who do. There is no need to feel guilty or alone. Find like-minded people to support you through your journey and formula-feed your baby in public with pride. Enjoy this precious time when you get to feed your baby while holding them closely. And remember that what matters most is having a healthy, happy, and thriving baby, parent, and family.

OTHER TOPICS FOR FORMULA-FEEDING FAMILIES

Information on the following can be found at the QR code:

- Is colic caused by bottle feeding or formula?
- Can I overfeed my formula-fed baby?
- Do formula-feeding babies cluster-feed?
- How do formula fed babies obtain antibodies?
- How can I ensure good dental hygiene for my formula-fed baby?
- How do I dry up my milk supply if I intend to only formula-feed?
- How and when do I wean my child from formula?

10

Combination Feeding

Combination breast milk and formula feeding, or combo feeding (CF), is perhaps the most common form of infant feeding in the world, yet the least talked about in educational resources. While most of the world's infants are breastfed, only a minority are *exclusively* breastfed to six months for various reasons, and even fewer to a year, leaving a significant portion of infants combo fed or formula fed.[1] While 58 percent of US families are breastfeeding at six months, only 27 percent are breastfeeding exclusively, meaning 31 percent of babies receive both formula and breast milk in their first year of life.[2]

Some blame the lack of community-based lactation support and other social barriers for low exclusive breastfeeding rates. Yet, this is not always the case, as we have learned. The data shows that more than 1 in 7 healthy mothers will have persistent milk supply problems even with intensive lactation support.[3] (If you include mothers who are older than thirty years, have BMI greater than 30 kg/m^2, or have medical problems, then insufficient milk supply is even more common.[4])

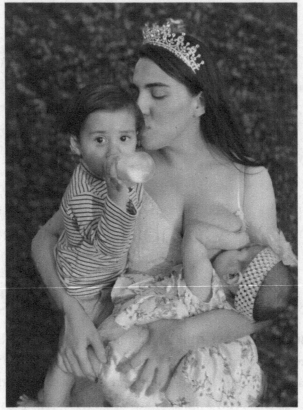

Sandra Stephany Lozoya breastfeeding and formula-feeding her babies

Even under ideal circumstances, supplementation is common. For example, in Norway, which at 99 percent has the highest rate of breastfeeding initiation in the industrialized world, as well as excellent parental leave policies, only 7 percent of babies are still exclusively breastfed at six months.[5] By four months, 33 percent are consuming some formula, and by six months, 43 percent are.

Parents combo-feed for many reasons. Some mothers start off intending to exclusively breastfeed but end up combo feeding when they find they have a partial milk supply, even with maximal effort and professional breastfeeding support. Others wish to have a partner feed formula at night. Some mothers choose to exclusively breastfeed and pump for several weeks while on maternity leave. Then, as they prepare for returning to work or other outside-the-home activities, they transition to combo-feeding or exclusive formula feeding (see "Weaning from Pumping" in chapter eight, page 222). Although all nursing parents should be provided workplace accommodations, some have jobs not conducive to pumping breaks (airline pilots, teachers, surgeons, trial attorneys, line cooks, and many others) or have employers who are not subject to this federal regulation. Still others choose to combo-feed from birth to weaning.

Common reasons for wanting to combo-feed include:

- to facilitate longer blocks of uninterrupted sleep for parents who are negatively affected by lack of sleep.
- to cope better with the stress of infant parenting.
- to allow mothers who are taking medications with limited safety research to minimize their infant's exposure.
- to allow some mothers to extend their time breastfeeding if exclusive breastfeeding is unsustainable for any reason.
- to ensure their baby will take both breast milk and formula by bottle before returning to work.
- to provide peace of mind if there is trauma from past breastfeeding problems or infant-feeding complications, and to prevent risk for subsequent babies.
- to allow partners to participate and have shared responsibility in infant feeding.
- to accommodate the mother's informed choice.

Support for those who combo-feed is important because mothers often report not breastfeeding as long as they had wanted to prenatally,[6] and there is almost no support for parents who choose to combo-feed. Combo-feeding parents often tell us that they would have appreciated being taught about combo feeding in their breastfeeding classes and that it might have helped them continue to breastfeed longer.

> I was never informed I could combo-feed, and if I knew it was a
> viable option, I would have tried, as a low-producing mother. I
> thought it was either breastfeeding or formula feeding. I regret
> not knowing this.
>
> —Heather Robertson

This chapter therefore focuses on filling these knowledge gaps and teaching how to sustain combination feeding while addressing its challenges. While the lactation research is replete with ideas on how to increase exclusive-breastfeeding rates, it is mostly silent on how to sustain breastfeeding while also supplementing with formula. Combination feeding is usually framed as a threat to sustained breastfeeding. While it can be *if* steps aren't taken to protect milk production and latching, successful combo feeding is not only possible but widely practiced. In fact, a 2019 study specifically shows that giving one formula feeding a day of 4 ounces or less, even in the first month, is perfectly compatible with continued breastfeeding,[7] not to mention three decades of global data showing that most breastfeeding mothers combo-feed, often for extended durations (up to two years or more).[8]

GRIEVING WHEN THINGS DON'T GO AS PLANNED

We want to acknowledge that mothers who need to combo-feed due to uncorrectable low supply often grieve the loss of exclusive breastfeeding. While combo feeding meets the baby's needs, it does not solve the mother's emotional pain over not having the breastfeeding experience she had imagined, especially if she believes that it's somehow her fault (untrue) or that formula is bad for her baby (also untrue). Even in ideal circumstances, having a partial milk supply is common.[9] Despite what others may say, combination feeding for partial-supply parents who wish to breastfeed is, in fact, "best." It often enables a mother to breastfeed for longer than she would with an unsustainable breastfeeding and pumping regimen that does not ultimately achieve a full supply.

HOW TO COMBO-FEED

There is no single "right" way to combo-feed, since each family determines what works best for them. Combo feeding comes in many forms, from mostly breastfeeding with occasional formula as needed, to mostly formula feeding but providing a small amount of human milk by breast or bottle. Some intend to combo-feed from the start; others simply play it by ear and do whatever works best. Think about your family's daily and weekly routine, then identify when your body makes the most milk and when supplemental formula feeding could work best. Every breastfeeding mother's body (and milk supply) responds differently to different combo-feeding regimens. Your baby will also have their own opinions about how and when they are fed. Trial and error are an important part of finding what combo-feeding method works best for you. If you find yourself struggling to make it work, we recommend working with a lactation consultant experienced in successful combo feeding.

Let's first review some fundamentals of milk production and how to avoid dwindling supply. With this knowledge, you should find it easier to start and keep combo-feeding as long as you and your baby want. The key factor in maintaining milk supply is regularly removing milk from the breasts. Your breasts' storage capacity determines how often they need to be drained to maintain supply. Mothers with a lower-than-average milk supply or who have lower storage capacity will likely need their breasts drained every two to three hours; those with higher milk supply have larger capacity and may be able to go four to five hours. Therefore, the most important rule of combo feeding is knowing your approximate storage capacity, then breastfeeding or pumping *before* your breasts become uncomfortably full. If you would like to experiment with stretching out pumping intervals, we recommend keeping track of your twenty-four-hour milk production for a week or so to confirm you are making the same amount.

While determining your combo-feeding regimen, remember the difference between normal fullness and *engorgement*. Normal fullness means your breasts are heavy, may be slightly uncomfortable, and may be leaking. In contrast, engorgement is very painful; your breasts feel warm and rock hard, and the skin is often shiny and lumpy. Tolerating some fullness may be necessary to reduce supply enough to enable combo-feeding, but do your best to avoid engorgement, as it increases the risk of milk stasis, plugged ducts, and mastitis.[10]

SAMPLE COMBO-FEEDING SCHEDULES

Each baby is different, and your feeding and pumping regimen should match your and the baby's needs. All babies should be fed according to hunger cues, not strict time schedules. Flexibility is key. Here are some possible approaches:[11]

KEY

BF: Direct breastfeeding
EM: Expressed milk
F: Formula
P: Pumping
PP: Power-pumping session

Temporary Supplementation Until Full Milk Supply Comes In

7 AM	10 AM	1 PM	4 PM	7 PM	10 PM	1 AM	4 AM
BF + F	BF + F	BF + F	BF + F	BF + F	BF + F	BF + F	BF + F

Delayed onset of lactogenesis II (DLII) is common and requires temporary supplementation, which can start as soon as you notice your baby is still hungry after breastfeeding. Some mothers with risk factors, insufficient glandular tissue, or a history of low milk supply may know they want to supplement or combo-feed from the very first meal, until their milk is in, to avoid feeding complications. (Note: Having a history of DLII or low supply does not mean you will have it again. Onset of lactogenesis II and milk supply vary with each pregnancy.)

Supplementation given *after* fully emptying both breasts at least every three hours allows for the stimulus needed to maximize milk supply. Once milk supply meets the infant's needs, you can stop supplementing and resume exclusive breastfeeding, if desired (see page 196).

Temporary supplementation does not *require* a breast pump, since the baby does the job of removing the milk. Also, you won't need to refrigerate, since any breast milk produced is directly fed to the baby. This may be useful in settings without access to breast pumps or refrigeration.

Temporary Supplementation When Baby Is Not Nursing Effectively at Birth

7 AM	10 AM	1 PM	4 PM	7 PM	10 PM	1 AM	4 AM
BF ± P after*	P + F	BF ± P after*	P + F	BF ± P after*	P + F	BF ± P after*	P + F

Pump after breastfeeding if the feeding is ineffective.

Early-term babies (37–39 weeks) may not be able to nurse effectively. In general, they are very sleepy and may latch on, take a few sucks, and fall back asleep. Breastfeeding them can be challenging because of their unpredictable energy levels, but one potential solution is to supplement in order to give them a break every other feeding and conserve their energy. Another is to limit breastfeeding sessions to ten minutes to conserve their energy for the next feeding. Both potential solutions reduce the need to triple-feed at every feeding (breastfeed, bottle-feed, and pump) until they are mature enough to breastfeed effectively.

Remember to breastfeed your baby on both sides. If a feeding is short or ineffective, pump afterward and feed your baby with the expressed milk obtained. If your baby is still exhibiting hunger cues after this, they likely need formula supplementation. Check with your doctor. Your next feeding will be with a bottle, which a partner can assist with while you pump to protect your milk supply. You can save the expressed milk for your next bottle feeding.

It is common for mothers to wonder how long their baby will be sleepy and not nurse effectively. Usually, once early babies reach their due date, they become more efficient nursers and have the stamina to nurse effectively at every feeding. A few babies will need more time to mature. Direct breast-feeding sessions can be increased as your baby matures and gains strength to nurse effectively.

Extended Combo Feeding from Birth

7 AM	10 AM	1 PM	4 PM	7 PM	10 PM	1 AM	4 AM
BF	BF	BF	F ± P	F ± P	BF	F	BF

Families who wish to combo-feed from birth can begin on the day of birth, even from the first feed. Others may pick a particular time to feed formula, like late afternoon when milk supply is lowest and/or the middle of the night to facilitate sleep. Partners can help with bottle feeds.

If your goal is to feed both breast milk and formula throughout the day and your breasts are full of more milk than you need, not pumping during formula feeding sessions will downregulate your milk production. Make sure to manage uncomfortable fullness with cold compresses, a supportive bra, and ibuprofen to reduce any discomfort and/or swelling; scan the QR code for more on managing engorgement.

Combo-Feeding While Facilitating a Five-Hour Block of Uninterrupted Sleep

7 AM	10 AM	1 PM	4 PM	7 PM	10 PM	10:30 PM– 3:30 AM	3:30 AM
BF	BF	BF	BF + F	BF + F	BF	SLEEP; partner feeds F at 1:30 AM	BF, then pump; or P for 10 minutes, then BF

As discussed in chapter eight, some nursing parents need an uninterrupted block of sleep due to psychological and medical conditions, or because extra sleep amid the intense demands of being a new parent will improve their quality of life. Getting five straight hours a night while a partner feeds a bottle of expressed milk or formula can help some continue to breastfeed instead of stopping altogether.

To help protect your milk supply and reduce breast fullness, it's important to fully express both breasts after you awaken from the five-hour block. You can breastfeed first, then pump. Or, if engorgement is painful or prevents latch, you can pump for five to ten minutes upon waking, then nurse to completely drain the breasts.

Breastfeeding While Giving Bottles During Times of Low Milk Production

7 AM	10 AM	1 PM	4 PM	7 PM	10 PM	1 AM	4 AM
BF	BF	BF	BF + F	BF + F	BF	BF	BF

Some parents, especially those with a partial milk supply, find the early evenings most difficult because babies are often fussy and nurse more frequently and longer. This is typically when milk production is at its lowest. Increased time and frequency of nursing (cluster feeding) can be normal in the evenings for two to three hours, but if your baby continues to appear hungry despite this, you can offer formula to satisfaction.

Some resources say that cluster feeding is essential for increasing milk supply. Whether this is true is unknown, given there are no studies.[12] But if your baby has been nursing for most of three hours and there is no more available milk, who gains from continued breastfeeding? There is no evidence that continuing to breastfeed while keeping a baby hungry for hours benefits moms, babies, or breastfeeding. Some have done this only to discover their child failed to thrive after weeks of effort.[13] Your baby deserves to be satisfied when they are hungry or thirsty.

Formula Feeding During Work Hours While Breastfeeding at Home

7 AM	10 AM	1 PM	4 PM	7 PM*	10 PM	1 AM	3 AM
BF	F	F	F	BF	BF	BF	BF

*Or upon arriving home.

Some parents are unable to pump during work hours but can breastfeed at home while a caretaker formula-feeds during the day. Note that not pumping at work can gradually diminish milk supply if breast fullness is prolonged (meaning it lasts more than five hours). However, some with large milk capacities may be still able to maintain their supply with this schedule.

Alternating Breastfeeding and Formula Throughout the Day

7 AM	10 AM	1 PM	4 PM	7 PM	10 PM	1 AM	4 AM	7 AM
B	F	B	F	B	F	B	F	B

Breastfeeding while formula-feeding every other feed may be an option for those with a larger milk storage capacity and a milk production rate that allows it. This routine allows for equal sharing of infant feeding and may be less demanding for mothers who are struggling with exclusive breastfeeding or pumping.

Alternating Pumping and Formula-Feeding Throughout the Day

7 AM	10 AM	1 PM	4 PM	7 PM	10 PM	1 AM	4 AM	7 AM
P + F	EM	P + F	EM	P + F	EM	P + F	EM	P + F

Mothers who cannot or do not wish to have their babies latch directly and who can maintain their supply with less frequent pumping are good candidates for this schedule. Families who want to share feeding responsibilities also may find this schedule desirable.

Pumping, Then Expressed Milk Feeding with Formula as Needed

7 AM	10 AM	1 PM	4 PM	7 PM	10 PM	1 AM	4 AM
P → EM	P → EM	P → EM	P → EM	P → EM + F	P → EM + F	P → EM	P → EM

Some mothers wish to see how much milk they are making before feeding it to their baby because of concerns about low milk supply or slow growth. They may use this information to know how much formula to supplement with or to feel reassured that their infant is getting enough milk.

Breastfeeding for "Dessert" After Bottle Feeding for Low-Supply Mothers

7 AM	10 AM	1 PM	4 PM	7 PM	10 PM	1 AM	4 AM
Partial F, then BF	Partial F, then BF	Partial F, then BF	Partial F, then BF	Partial F, then BF	Partial F, then BF	Partial F, then BF	Partial F, then BF

For some combo-fed babies, breastfeeding before the bottle (as recommended to ensure adequate breast stimulation) does not work. In cases of very low supply, a hungry baby can get easily frustrated when milk does not flow from the breast as quickly as they want. This negative association can cause breast refusal. Offering the bottle first with an approximate volume of formula that they typically get after nursing, then finishing at the breast, is a strategy that some combo-feeding mothers use to help their babies enjoy and want to continue breastfeeding. This may seem counter-intuitive, but it allows them to associate fullness with the breast instead of the bottle, and mothers often find this a more enjoyable way to conclude the feeding.[14]

This method can be used short term or long term. We have worked with mothers who nursed their babies for two-plus years using this approach, because many babies nurse for comfort, not just for food. Scan the QR code to learn more.

BREASTFEEDING WHILE USING A SUPPLEMENTAL NURSING SYSTEM FOR FEEDING FORMULA

A supplemental nursing system (SNS) is a tool that allows a parent to supplement formula to their infant from a reservoir through a tube taped to the nipple. Common reasons for using an SNS include maintaining direct breastfeeding when supplementation is needed, preventing bottle preference, and providing the stimulation to increase milk supply (when paired with effective latch and frequent milk expression).

Mothers with chronic low supply can use an SNS to supplement at the breast instead of a bottle either exclusively if they want, or just occasionally in order to prevent bottle preference (see chapter eleven), as supplementing with an SNS maintains the association of milk coming from the breast no matter how much milk is produced. This is particularly helpful for those with very limited supply, as they are at highest risk of losing the direct nursing relationship and, subsequently, what milk supply they have. Many with low milk supply credit an SNS with saving their breastfeeding experience, allowing them to breastfeed for much longer than with a previous baby.

Not all nursing parents like using an SNS, however. Some find them awkward and cumbersome. Some don't want the added burden of cleaning and sterilizing SNS parts. Many babies continue nursing directly without it, for comfort and the taste of breast milk, while getting formula from a bottle instead. If your baby won't latch with the SNS or you don't like the SNS, bottles are always an option.

MANAGING COMMON CHALLENGES IN COMBINATION FEEDING

Combination feeding requires managing both breastfeeding and formula-feeding challenges, in addition to other complications unique to combination feeding. These include managing oversupply in the beginning, maintaining your infant's interest in the breast *and* the bottle, and maintaining your desired milk supply.

Breast Engorgement While Reducing a Full Supply

As the full milk supply comes in, those who plan to combo-feed from the start may find they temporarily have more milk than they need and want to take steps to reduce their supply. To begin reducing your milk supply, you can try either or both of the methods below, depending on your comfort.

Method 1: Skip one breastfeeding or pumping session per day for four to seven days until your breasts have adjusted, as indicated by less engorgement. You can skip another session per day for another four to seven days until your breasts adjust again. Continue repeating this pattern until your pumping frequency and milk supply are at your desired level.

Some may reach their desired level of supply quickly, while others may require longer due to discomfort and/or a large milk supply. Note: If at any time your breasts are very uncomfortable during weaning, you may express for two or three minutes for relief without compromising your efforts to reduce your supply. Some breasts may leak when full.

Method 2: Gradually reduce the number of minutes you are pumping per session (from 15 to 12 minutes, then 12 to 10 minutes, and so on) every four to seven days. This is useful for nursing parents who have a history of mastitis and want to prevent it or for those who want a slower, more controlled weaning process. It will likely take longer than Method 1, but your comfort level is important, too.

Remember to slow down or back off of reducing the number of breast-feeding or pumping sessions or your pumping duration if it's causing pain from engorgement.

Once your milk supply reaches a level that meets your baby's requirement without discomfort from engorgement, then breastfeeding and/or pumping at the same frequency is likely to maintain your supply.

Formula Refusal When Transitioning from Exclusive Breastfeeding to Combo Feeding

If your baby has been exclusively breastfeeding and is transitioning to CF, they may initially refuse formula. It may be the bottle, the taste of the formula, or both.

If you haven't yet introduced a bottle, first offer the baby expressed milk by bottle. If they refuse it, try leaving your home and having another family member give it. The presence of your baby's preferred method of feeding (your breasts) may hinder acceptance of the bottle.

Once your baby accepts expressed milk in a bottle, if they still refuse the formula bottle, we suggest the following. Start with a small bottle so, if they reject it, waste is minimized. Start by mixing 1 ounce (30 mL) of breast milk and half a teaspoon (2.5 mL) of prepared formula. Offer it to your baby. Once your baby reliably takes the mixed bottle, gradually increase the amount of formula and decrease the amount of breast milk in the bottle (20 mL breast milk and 5 mL formula, and so on).

If this doesn't work, you can also try a different formula.

Breast or Bottle Refusal

In general, babies adapt well to switching between bottle and breastfeeding if the bottle is offered within two or three weeks after birth. Sometimes, though, even if they have been taking both, babies can develop a preference for one or the other. This is challenging for parents who want to do both. Here are some helpful tips if babies begin to prefer one. Remember, the goal is to keep both feeding experiences equally pleasant, satisfying, and engaging.

Tips for Avoiding Breast Refusal

- Rapid flow from overactive letdown can be unpleasant for your baby. If you suspect this is the issue, try pumping for five to ten minutes before feeding to help reduce the flow.
- If milk supply is limited and slow flow is frustrating your baby, try the breastfeeding-for-dessert method (page 261).
- If breastfeeding latch is difficult, work with a lactation consultant and/or use a nipple shield.

Tips for Avoiding Bottle Refusal

- If your baby is refusing previously pumped milk, make sure your breast milk has not gone bad. Try tasting it. It should be slightly sweet with no off-putting flavor.
- If your baby is collapsing the bottle nipple, try switching to a nipple with increased flow rate (commonly needed around 3 months of age).

- Your baby may not like the shape of the nipple. If they are not latching deeply, try a narrower-shaped nipple. If they are gagging, try a smaller preemie or wide-based nipple.
- If your baby tends to cry during or after feeds, they may be swallowing too much air, and a (different) vented bottle system may help.

HOW TO MATCH A BOTTLE NIPPLE'S FLOW WITH YOUR OWN NIPPLE'S FLOW

Most CF babies switch easily between breast and bottle until weaning. Some can develop a preference for one method. If this becomes a concern, you can try to match the flow rate of their bottle's nipple with your own.

1. Time an average breastfeeding session either in the late morning or early afternoon. Avoid using the first feeding of the day or the late afternoon, as these sessions are typically the fastest- and slowest-flow feeds, respectively.
2. Start with a slow-flow nipple (labeled as newborn, level 1, or 0 month).
3. The next day, instead of directly breastfeeding at this same time, pump and feed expressed milk or formula through the nipple you are testing, while timing the session.
4. The amount of time spent feeding by bottle should be about the same as the time breastfeeding directly. If the bottle-feeding session is *longer* than breastfeeding, buy a higher-flow-rate nipple; if the bottle feeding is *shorter*, try a lower-flow-rate nipple.

Supporting Ongoing Milk Production

At some point, your baby may require more milk than they are getting from their current combo-feeding regimen. This additional milk can be breast milk or formula, depending on your preference. If you wish to meet this increased need with breast milk, you can do so with additional breast-feeding, pumping, and/or feeding your stored breast milk. If your baby is hungry after their usual supplemental bottle, try offering the breast again to stimulate increased milk production (for around 10 minutes, or as long as your baby is willing) before giving them additional supplemental milk to satisfaction. Otherwise, instead of additional breastfeeding, you can simply pump for ten minutes.

If your milk supply does not increase after a week of this, or if you just want to use formula to meet their increased need, then offer formula to satisfaction after nursing. So long as you are expressing milk at the same frequency and duration, your milk supply should stay the same.

Remember to balance increased time nursing and pumping with other considerations, such as protecting your nipples from overuse, having time to do other things like sleeping and enjoying your family, and protecting your mental health. Some mothers find themselves in an ever-increasing cycle of nursing and pumping that slowly takes over all other aspects of their life. Set healthy limits for yourself and decide what amount of breastfeeding, pumping, and formula feeding allows your whole family to thrive.

"THE BEST OF BOTH WORLDS"

Combination feeding can be very rewarding. Parents who have done it describe it as "the best of both worlds." While many mothers want to breast-feed, feeding problems are common, as are the social and economic barriers that compound them. Parents are commonly given advice that presents for-mula as less than ideal, risky, and competing against breastfeeding, rather than being a tool that can help sustain it. This leaves mothers who combo-feed feeling like the feeding regimen that best fits their bodies and their babies is a problem that needs fixing rather than a healthy solution.

If the breastfeeding and pumping regimen recommended for low milk supply doesn't produce the desired result of a full supply, it can lead to negative self-image, depression, and sometimes a poorly growing child. Ironically, the very regimen used to promote breastfeeding in this scenario may be what ultimately ends it.

Remember, combo feeding has been done for generations and is the most common method of infant feeding around the world. If you find that combo feeding best meets your and your baby's needs, then you are giving your child the best. Be proud and celebrate it.

11

Bottle Feeding with Breast Milk or Formula

Bottles are a staple of infant feeding, used by families who formula-feed, combination-feed, and exclusively feed breast milk alike. So why do we have a whole chapter dedicated to bottle feeding? Because bottle feeding—just like breastfeeding—is a complex interaction between the parent, baby, and feeding source, and too few resources provide comprehensive bottle-feeding information using the latest scientific research. As a result, few parents are aware that there is a body of knowledge about bottle feeding that can inform their decision making. Without this information, it can be difficult to know what is scientifically validated and what is pure conjecture.

For instance, many parents are taught that bottle-fed infants don't have to work as hard as breastfed babies to get milk, so they are prone to getting overfed and therefore at higher risk of obesity, which has not been established (see chapter three).[1] While it is possible to overfeed bottle-fed babies, few parents know that *how* you bottle-feed and respond to your baby's cues

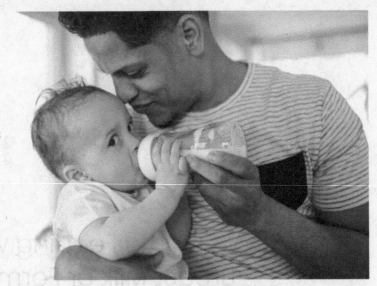

Bottle feeding with optimal upright positioning

can determine whether they are overfed, which may in turn affect future eating habits. We will discuss this in full.

Parents are frequently taught that bottle feeding and breastfeeding are distinctly different in other ways, too, and that special equipment and techniques are necessary to help breastfed babies bottle-feed "like they are breastfeeding."[2] Neither claim is supported by research. This has led to the marketing of expensive "just like breastfeeding" bottles and nipples that have questionable or unproven benefits. As a 2020 literature review by Kotowski et al. found:

> The majority of the studies concluded that healthy term bottle-feeding infants use similar tongue and jaw movements compared with breastfeeding infants when obtaining milk during a feed.[3]

Still, despite these similarities, bottle feeding has distinct features that can be adjusted to best fit the baby's needs, which this chapter explains.

THE MECHANICS OF MILK INTAKE

Term infants are born with feeding reflexes like rooting, where they turn their head toward a touch on the face, which helps them locate human and bottle nipples alike. Infants' mouths will also open if a nipple touches their lower lip. And as soon as the nipple touches the roof of their mouth, the sucking reflex activates. The sucking reflex involves three parts: (1) sucking, (2) swallowing, and (3) breathing. (This is referred to by speech therapists as SSB.) The mouth, jaw, and tongue are all used to generate the suction and compression needed to transfer milk.

Milk intake by bottle is affected by how babies are positioned, as gravity can increase the flow of milk in a reclined or flat position. Intake is also affected by the rate of milk flow through the nipple; the nipple's shape, length, and compressibility; whether the nipple or bottle is vented; and other features, like whether a collapsible bag is used. Most term infants have no problems with bottle feeding, but some preterm infants need additional interventions to bottle-feed given their decreased strength and coordination. Check with their doctor.

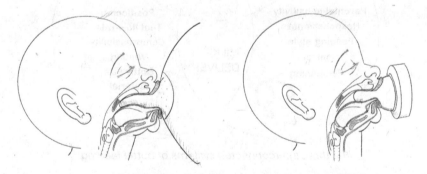

Side-by-side comparison of the latch of a breastfeeding baby and bottle-feeding baby; they are very similar.

THE THREE INTERCONNECTED
SYSTEMS OF BOTTLE FEEDING

Kotowski et al.'s review identified three interconnected systems that affect bottle feeding, all of which must work together to provide optimal outcomes for a baby. Put simply, they are:

1. **The bottle**—including the nipple and its features.
2. **The baby**—their feeding reflexes, sucking pattern, and positioning.
3. **The parent**—how they recognize and respond to infant cues.

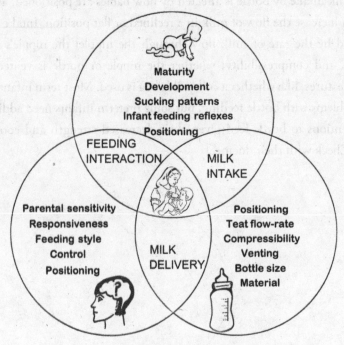

The three interconnected systems of bottle feeding

These three systems interact to affect a baby's bottle-feeding experience. Parents can affect milk delivery by choosing different nipple flow rates and bottle designs, for instance. The baby's milk intake can be affected by their sucking pattern and the bottle's design. The parent and the baby's feeding interaction and positioning during bottle feeding can affect infant self-regulation of milk intake, possible future eating habits, and health outcomes. Among these important interactions is responsive feeding, a baby-led form of feeding that relies on parents recognizing and responding to infant hunger and satisfaction cues to start and stop feeds, which is recommended by health organizations for bottle-fed and breastfed infants alike.[4]

There are feeding factors parents cannot control, like a baby's mouth anatomy or sucking pattern and strength. However, parents can significantly affect several factors: (1) nipple and bottle selection, (2) feeding position, and (3) responsive feeding.

Nipple and Bottle Selection

Choosing bottles and nipples for your baby can be overwhelming, thanks to so many options, marketing taglines, and "expert" opinions on the matter. But there is no such thing as one "best" baby bottle or nipple because babies have unique oral anatomy and sucking mechanics. Most babies do fine with whatever they are given, but some require adjustments to the bottle or nipple to have the most comfortable experience. Problems that can be solved by changing the bottle or nipple include excessive gas, frustration with slow or fast flow, gagging, and poor latch, to name a few. It may take some experimentation to find the right nipple for your baby, but paying attention to the following factors can help you find the right one.

1. NIPPLE FLOW RATE

Flow rate is one of the most important considerations in choosing a nipple for babies. It determines how well they can regulate the amount of milk they take with each swallow. While a slow-flow nipple is recommended for newborns, flow needs in older babies can vary.

Fortunately, independent research has provided information on nipple flow rates to help parents select the best nipple for their baby, at any age.[5] If the flow rate is too high, babies can struggle to manage flow and have stressful feedings. If it is too low, babies can become frustrated and burn more energy working to extract milk.

Keep in mind that it's important to experiment, especially if a nipple you choose has not been tested by researchers, as some labeled "slow flow" may actually flow more quickly than a baby can tolerate.

HOW TO KNOW IF A NIPPLE'S FLOW RATE IS RIGHT FOR YOUR BABY

Feeds that are shorter or longer than the typical fifteen-to-twenty-minute feeding may indicate too fast or too slow a nipple flow, respectively.[6] If your baby seems easily frustrated while feeding, is regularly collapsing the nipple or having to release the nipple every few sucks, crying, or maybe even refusing the bottle if combination-feeding, your nipple flow rate may be too slow, and you may need to select a higher-flow-rate nipple. If your baby has milk flowing out of the sides of their mouth, is sputtering or choking on the flow, or refusing the bottle, the nipple flow is too fast.

For breastfeeding families who use bottles, it is important to know that some infants can develop preference for the bottle over the breast if the former has an easier or faster flow of milk. Some babies can reject the bottle and prefer the breast, due to bottle flow being too slow or too fast, or dislike for nipple shape, length, or material. Matching the bottle nipple's flow rate with your breasts' nipple flow rate is one option that may help maintain equal preference (see page 266).

---

2. NIPPLE SHAPE AND LENGTH

There are five main categories of nipples:

1. **Traditional or narrow-necked nipples,** which fit better into smaller mouths and allow for a deeper latch than other nipples.
2. **Wide-based nipples,** which are often marketed as "similar to the breast" due to their shape: wider at the base of the nipple with a shorter nipple length. However, they don't stretch like breasts and

have an abrupt change in slope that can limit effective suction due to shallow latch.

3. **Medium-neck nipples**, which provide a compromise between narrow-necked and wide-based nipples.

4. **Orthodontic nipples**, lipstick-shaped nipples marketed as reducing the risk of misaligned teeth. These may limit deep latch and change sucking patterns, leading to sore nipples for parents who also nurse. A 2016 systematic review found insufficient evidence that these were effective at reducing dental issues when compared to narrow-neck nipples.[7]

5. **Preemie nipples**, which are designed to be narrow, very soft, and flexible, with a very slow milk flow.

There are also different nipple lengths. Infants with sensitive gag reflexes may benefit from shorter nipples, and those who have trouble getting a good latch may benefit from longer nipples.

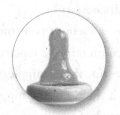
Narrow neck, narrow base premie nipple

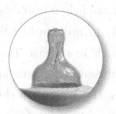
Traditional narrow neck, medium-based nipple

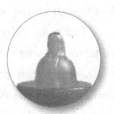
Gradual-slope, medium-based nipple

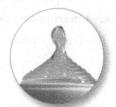
Orthodontic, wide-based nipple

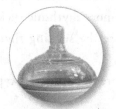
Narrow neck, wide-based nipple

Types of nipples

3. NIPPLE COMPRESSIBILITY

Nipples are usually made from either latex or silicone. Latex nipples are softer and more elastic than silicone, but they must be replaced as often as every two months as they break down sooner and become sticky. Some babies can develop an allergy to latex nipples, and for this reason, many parents choose silicone nipples. Silicone nipples also last longer (usually three months) and collapse less during feeding.

A bottle nipple that is soft and flexible helps a baby maintain the latch through the duration of the feeding, because it is easier to pull, stretch, and compress to transfer milk efficiently and comfortably. A baby with a powerful suck may feed better with a nipple that is more rigid and resists compression, preventing nipple collapse.

4. VENTING

Most infants swallow some air during bottle feeding, but some either swallow more or are more sensitive to the amount they swallow. Removing bubbles through vented bottles can help minimize gas discomfort.[8]

When your baby sucks in milk from a bottle, a vacuum is formed inside, unlike when they suck on a breast. This vacuum must be replaced by air, which can enter through the hole at the tip of the nipple or another hole in the system. If air comes in through the tip of the nipple or anywhere under the milk, the air must pass through the milk, causing bubbles. Using a vented bottle system provides a way for air to displace this vacuum while minimizing mixture of air with milk. This reduces the amount of air swallowed and discomfort from gas. The venting also allows for more rhythmic sucking and fewer interruptions during feeding, because the sucking rhythm can be sustained without collapsing the nipple.

There are three different types of vents:

1. **Nipple vents** are holes located at the base of the nipple. Since the vents are submerged by the milk, the air bubbles go through the milk, increasing the amount of air the baby swallows.

2. **Straw vents** use straws, located by vents at the base of the nipple, to capture the air and direct it to the bottom of the bottle to prevent air mixture.

3. **Bottom-of-bottle venting valves** are removable, one-way silicone valves located at the bottom of the bottle that allow air to be drawn in above the milk line, thus preventing mixture.

The latter two have more parts to clean but are more effective for infants with gas discomfort.

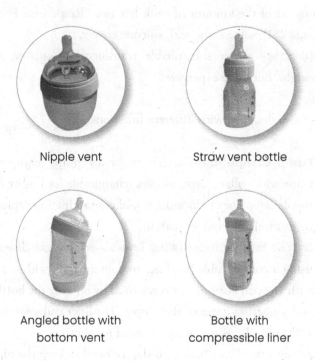

Nipple vent   Straw vent bottle

Angled bottle with   Bottle with
bottom vent   compressible liner

Types of vents

5. BOTTLES

Various types of bottles are available. All can handle temperatures needed for sterilization and are all BPA free. (BPA is an endocrine disruptor that can interfere with growth and reproductive development.)[9] Aside from differences in material and durability, bottles can have different features important for infant health and comfort.

Bottles are usually made from one of four materials:

1. **Plastic bottles**—the most common and least expensive; light, translucent, and durable.
2. **Glass**—recyclable and transparent, but heavy and slippery when wet and breakable if dropped; silicone covers can improve grip and reduce breakage.
3. **Stainless steel**—lightweight, and unbreakable; opaque, which may encourage parents to watch babies' hunger/fullness cues instead of the amount of milk left (see "Responsive Feeding" on page 281); some come with silicone covers.
4. **Silicone**—newer, soft, pliable, translucent to opaque, and lightweight, but more expensive.

Bottles are also designed with different functions:

- **Pump compatible**—attach to breast pump equipment, and come with collars, caps, nipples (changeable for higher flow), and nipple caps. They reduce the risk of contaminating expressed milk by minimizing contact with it.
- **Bottles with compressible liners**—reduce gas discomfort by using a compressible bag liner to contain milk within a chamber with an open bottom. Air is removed by holding the bottle upright and squeezing it out of the nipple. The liner collapses as the baby sucks in milk, eliminating the need for venting.
- **Angled bottles**—have a 30-degree bend to keep the nipple filled with milk while feeding a baby upright; also has a vented bottom to reduce air mixture and gas discomfort.

Scan the QR code for more detail on each type of bottle.

Feeding Position

Recent research has also found that how you position babies while bottle feeding makes a difference in developing ear and respiratory infections. A clinical trial conducted in Israel found that counseling parents who bottle-feed their babies with formula or breast milk to do so with the baby's head and torso in an upright, 90-degree position dramatically reduced rates of respiratory infections and related conditions.[10] Researchers randomly assigned participating pediatric clinics to the intervention group (counseling on upright positioning) versus control (no counseling), confirmed that the counseling was effective at changing bottle-feeding practices, and then looked at the rates of different common childhood illnesses in the month prior to the study and in the year following, including:

- ear infections (otitis media) or ear fluid (serous otitis media).
- respiratory conditions, such as a persistent cough, wheezing, bronchitis, or pneumonia.
- prolonged fever episodes lasting three days or more.
- antibiotic use.
- inhaled bronchodilator use (for wheezing).

At the beginning of the study, parent reports of these illnesses were similar. The parents were surveyed again after three, six, nine, and twelve months, and the investigators found that rates of illness in all five categories had dropped significantly in the upright bottle-feeding group. Rates of respiratory infections dropped by 12–46 percent across the four surveyed time points, ear infections by 15–58 percent, prolonged fever by 27–68 percent, inhaler use by 5–48 percent, and antibiotic use by 26–52 percent. The differences seemed to diminish at twelve months, when most infants sit upright on their own. The only other significant factor that predicted development of these illnesses was daycare use.

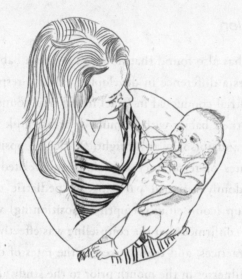

Recommended upright position for bottle feeding

Other studies have found that bottle feeding in a supine (lying down) or semi-supine (reclined) position can lead to formula entering the middle ear through the Eustachian tubes, which connect the oral cavity to the ear.[11] Researchers and physicians think this may contribute to higher rates of middle ear infections in bottle-fed babies, whether they are fed breast milk or formula. It is also possible that supine positioning can lead to infants breathing milk into the lungs, which increases the risk of pneumonia. These findings are incredibly important, as they suggest that increased ear and respiratory illnesses commonly associated with bottle and formula feeding may be reduced simply by bottle-feeding in an upright position.

Positioning a baby as upright as possible also helps them to control the flow of milk out of the nipple through sucking, rather than receiving milk passively through gravity. Researchers believe this ability to control milk intake is important in helping infants learn to recognize sensations of hunger and satisfaction, which is thought in turn to lead to healthier eating patterns as toddlers and adults.

Scan the QR code for images and descriptions of different ways to hold your baby upright from the newborn stage to around six months.

Responsive Feeding

How much milk a baby takes can be affected by their interaction with the person feeding them. Research has shown that an infant's ability to self-regulate their milk intake is affected by who is "in control" of the feeding, the parent or the infant. Some parents worry about overfeeding and may encourage lower intake. Others worry that their baby won't eat enough and encourage continued feeding even after their infants are full. If parents strongly lead the feeding interaction, the child can underfeed or overfeed, both of which are thought to increase the risk of unhealthy eating habits.

The solution to both problems is *responsive feeding*, which the AAP and global infant-feeding guidelines recommend for reducing overfeeding and underfeeding of infants, whether they are fed with formula or human milk.[12] This technique requires the feeding person to closely follow the baby's feeding cues and to stop once they show signs of satisfaction.

This is very different from a popular bottle-feeding technique, supported by no evidence, known as *paced feeding*, a method that requires parent-led interruptions even during active feeding. These interruptions supposedly teach a baby to not overeat by forcing them to pause feeding every three to five swallows, then stopping when they are full.[13] Paced feeding is touted as the best way to prevent overfeeding, but instead it can discourage learning self-regulation and unnecessarily frustrate the baby. It can also cause a parent to focus on the technique rather than the important parent–infant interactions that promote responsiveness and bonding. Scan the QR code to learn more about paced feeding.

Babies' nutritional and fluid needs vary throughout the day and fluctuate during growth spurts, and bottle-feeding routines that offer the same amount of milk at the same time intervals can impair an infant's ability to self-regulate feeding.[14] Studies have found that when parents could not see or feel the amount of milk they had in a bottle, they were more attentive to their infant's signs of satisfaction, which resulted in more infant-led feeding.[15] In contrast, parents who were distracted by watching the milk in the bottle could miss their baby's cues, which can lead to under- or overfeeding.

Responsive feeding addresses the variation in an infant's nutritional needs by allowing them to control the timing and the amount they receive throughout the day. And, by using tools that force parents to rely on their infants' cues, rather than watching how much milk is left in the bottle, they can learn to recognize even subtle cues so they can get better at baby-led feeding.

BABIES WITH UNCLEAR HUNGER AND FULLNESS CUES

Some babies do not provide clear hunger and fullness cues, which can make responsive feeding more difficult. In such cases, it can be easy to overfeed or underfeed. Calculating the expected calorie needs for their weight (see page 153) and following their growth closely with their doctor will help prevent over- or undernutrition. Cue recognition can improve over time as the baby learns to provide clearer cues and parents learn to recognize more subtle ones.

HOW TO BOTTLE-FEED RESPONSIVELY[16]

The steps of responsive feeding are easy, but require parents to remain present and focused on their baby, which in our modern life can be difficult. Finding a quiet place without distractions like smartphones and televisions can be helpful.

1. Place your baby in the upright position of your choice.
2. Offer them the bottle by touching the nipple to their upper lip to elicit a gaping reflex.

3. As soon as your baby opens their mouth, angle the bottle to ensure the nipple is completely filled with milk. When your baby latches, they will begin sucking.

4. Allow your baby to take the lead, watching for cues of engagement or disengagement (see box below).

5. End the feeding once your baby shows signs of satisfaction.

Engagement Cues ("I'm hungry")	Disengagement Cues ("I'm full")
• Holding your gaze • Opening mouth • Putting hands in or near the mouth • Sucking sounds • Cycling through the suck–swallow–breathe pattern smoothly, with few interruptions	• Arching back, turning head, or leaning away • Crying • Falling asleep • Looking away • Pushing bottle away • Waving arm(s) • Negative facial expressions • Biting, chewing on, or spitting out nipple • Gagging, coughing, or choking • Spitting up

CLEANING AND STORING BABY BOTTLES AND NIPPLES

As important as our bottle-feeding technique is, we also need to make sure the bottles and nipples are free of harmful bacteria. Preventing contamination of human milk and formula is critically important to infant health and requires careful attention to all the steps needed to achieve it. This is particularly important for premature and medically fragile infants. (The following includes recommendations from the CDC, but check their guidelines periodically, as they are continually updated.[17]) As with pump parts, all items must be separated and cleaned after each use, including bottles, nipples, rings, and caps.[18]

To Clean Without a Dishwasher

1. Wash your hands.
2. Fill a clean basin used only for infant-feeding items with hot water and plain dish soap.
3. Take apart the bottle parts, rinse them, and put them in the basin.
4. Brush pieces thoroughly with a dedicated bottle brush and squeeze water through the nipple holes.
5. Rinse items, including the brush and basin, which should be air dried.
6. Feeding items can then be sanitized by boiling or steaming.
   - If boiling, submerge parts in a pot of boiling water for five minutes. Remove them using clean tongs and air-dry them on a clean paper towel.
   - If steaming, you can use commercially available microwavable steaming bags or bottle-steaming systems. Follow the manufacturer's instructions.

To Clean with a Dishwasher

1. Place items directly into the top rack, with nipples, caps, and screw rings in a dedicated closed basket to keep them contained during washing.
2. Use the sanitizing setting and heated drying.
3. Wash your hands before removing items from the dishwasher.
4. If additional drying is needed, let the items air-dry on a clean paper towel.

Once all the equipment is dry, wash your hands and put the pieces back together, including the cap to keep the nipple clean. Store all items, including your brush and basin (if applicable), in a cabinet only used for cleaning infant-feeding items. Make sure to replace any parts that show signs of wear and tear.

INTRODUCING THE BOTTLE IN BREASTFED INFANTS

There is one last bottle-feeding topic we need to discuss: introducing the bottle. Bottle refusal in breastfed infants is a common problem that can inconvenience any nursing mother wishing to spend more than a few hours away from her infant. Families are usually advised to wait on introducing a bottle until four to six weeks, until breastfeeding is established, to avoid nipple confusion. But research suggests that delaying bottle introduction may also lead to bottle refusal. In 2020, a UK study found that families experiencing bottle refusal had introduced the bottle, on average, at eight weeks, suggesting that waiting longer to introduce a bottle may increase the risk of refusal.[19]

Introducing the bottle to a previously breastfed-only baby can be difficult. The method for addressing bottle refusal in the above study that had the highest success rate was stopping breastfeeding altogether for those who intended to do so (see below). But for families who wish to continue breastfeeding while also using a bottle as needed, this method is not an option. The study found that other methods were helpful, but unfortunately, had lower success rates.

Methods for Addressing Bottle Refusal

Method	Success rate (%)
"Cold turkey" (complete cessation of breastfeeding)	42.4%
Partner/family fed the baby	21.1%
Used a cup (instead of a bottle)	19.2%
Used different bottles/nipples	15.4%
Used expressed breast milk in a bottle	12.8%
Gave bottle only when their baby was hungry	10.4%
Tried different formula milks	8.3%
Gave bottle only when their baby was not hungry	5.6%

What this study suggests is that for breastfeeding families who will need or want to bottle-feed expressed breast milk (or formula, if you need or want to combo-feed or previously used an SNS), introducing the bottle as early as possible and on a daily basis may help prevent bottle refusal. Unfortunately, there is no research to specify how early and how often to introduce the bottle to prevent refusal. For those concerned about early bottle introduction interfering with breastfeeding, no research has shown that the use of bottles with nipples to feed expressed breast milk interferes with breastfeeding, according to a WHO expert panel.[20] So long as you are breastfeeding and removing milk from the breasts frequently and adequately, research supports that you should not worry about bottle feeding interfering with breastfeeding.

BOTTLE FEEDING IS IMPORTANT, TOO

Bottle feeding has been essential to infant feeding since ancient times, and almost every household today relies on bottle feeding to nourish their babies, whether those bottles hold formula or breastmilk. Despite popular beliefs that bottle feeding is inferior to breastfeeding, research has shown that families can bottle-feed their babies with confidence. Upright bottle feeding has been shown to help reduce common infant respiratory infections. Responsive bottle feeding has been shown to promote optimal infant milk intake and may help babies develop healthy future eating habits. In addition, responsive feeding can improve parent awareness of infant cues, paving the way for healthier communication overall between a parent and their baby.

Infant feeding can be challenging, whatever the method, and it takes time and patience. But with the use of optimal bottle-feeding methods, it is more than possible for bottle-feeding families to provide a healthy and positive feeding experience for their babies.

OTHER TOPICS FOR BOTTLE-FEEDING FAMILIES

Information on the following and more can be found at the QR code below:

- Different bottle-feeding positioning for different age babies
- Infographics on bottle-feeding mechanics

TOPICS FOR FAMILIES WITH SPECIAL FEEDING NEEDS

Information on the following and more can be found at the QR code below:

- Feeding newborns who are premature or have other medical conditions
- Pumping schedules for parents pumping for premature infants in the NICU
- Tube feeding

12

Honoring All Families and All Forms of Safe Infant Feeding

Having a baby is a life-changing experience, the magnitude of which is impossible to comprehend until you experience it. Going from being completely independent to being responsible for a tiny person is the biggest change that many people face. If there is ever a time when you need kindness, support, and encouragement, it is now. Please know that you are doing one of the hardest jobs in the world, and if you are providing love, care, and healthy nourishment to your baby, you are parenting correctly.

Making feeding decisions is not as simple as picking between cloth and disposable diapers or choosing a stroller. Many parents think they will feed a certain way, only to find that it does not work for reasons they couldn't have predicted. Every parent has different life circumstances and biology, and even those with the best healthcare and unlimited resources are not immune to infant-feeding problems. Babies also have their own special circumstances like milk intolerances and anatomical variations. All of this means there is no single "best" form of infant feeding, despite what parents are told. To say there is only one "best" ignores the reality of this diversity, to the detriment of babies and families.

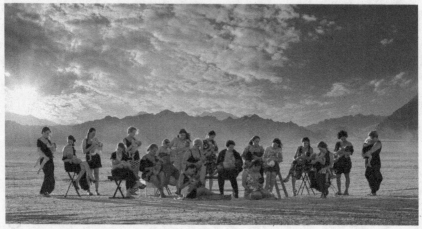

Fed Is Best Photo Shoot, 2018

Healthcare professionals *must* be able to offer evidence-based, noncommercial, and nonideological infant-feeding information that is inclusive, so that families can make choices that work best for them. *Every* new family needs and deserves support, whether they intend or need to breastfeed, combo-feed, or formula-feed.

THIS IS OUR MESSAGE IN A NUTSHELL

If you are breastfeeding: Your milk is an excellent source of nutrition and valuable in any amount you can and wish to provide. You should be able to nurse your babies anytime, anywhere, and be treated with respect. You deserve support and accommodations for breastfeeding from your employers, health providers, and society. You deserve accurate information on your child's nutrition. You and your baby are in charge of how much and how long you breastfeed.

If you are formula-feeding: You deserve access to formula that is safe, nutritious, and affordable. You should be able to bottle-feed your babies anytime, anywhere, and be treated with respect. Scientists have worked to design formula to be as close to breast milk as possible, making it an excellent source of nutrition. You and your baby can bond as deeply while bottle-feeding as you would while breastfeeding. You deserve accurate information unbiased by commercial interests or ideology.

If your child has special feeding needs: Your child's feeding should receive the same careful attention and affordability as every other form of feeding. Science has enabled us to protect the lives of the most vulnerable. Your child's feeding is equally important and should be celebrated.

If you are a healthcare provider who works with new families: You may be doing the best you can while being stuck between your clinical judgment and hospital policies that don't work for every family. You may have cared for babies who were either served poorly or harmed by the current guidelines. You may have been taught information that is outdated or wrong, and that is not your fault. If you are a lactation consultant, we celebrate your dedication to helping families breastfeed and welcome you to use our resources to ensure safe and sufficient breastfeeding for every baby. We know that all of the medical and other professionals involved in infant care—pediatricians, family physicians, obstetricians, nurse midwives, registered nurses, lactation consultants, dieticians, daycare providers, speech therapists, and more—care deeply about children and feeding them in a way that is safe, optimal, and ensures the best possible future. We must learn from mistakes already made, not just by individuals but in clinical guidelines and global health recommendations. We must evolve in response to what scientific evidence reveals, think critically about how it affects our patients' lives, and be willing to question, adjust, or even abandon beliefs that are causing harm, no matter how cherished those beliefs may be. We must demand change from hospitals and health policy makers when the standards are failing to protect and promote *optimal infant health.*

Pediatricians, other doctors, nurses, lactation consultants, and parents have all been warning us about the problems with the current guidelines: publishing letters, case reports, news articles, books, and research on infants harmed by rigid adherence to the exclusive breastfeeding policy for decades.[1] They have watched countless parents diligently try to meet this standard, wanting the best for their baby, only to return with a dehydrated, jaundiced, and starved infant. Researchers have been studying the harms of feeding complications, painstakingly measuring developmental outcomes and trying to determine the thresholds that define safe and unsafe. They have fiercely debated what those thresholds should be. We must respond by changing policies in response to what they uncover.

Almost every infant-feeding complication can be prevented if we listen to and believe our patients, examine them, measure objective markers of feeding, and *fully feed babies*. There is something seriously wrong when healthy newborns are being hospitalized for not getting enough milk. There is also something seriously wrong when mothers are developing depression and even thoughts of suicide because they feel pressured to feed their infants in only one way.[2] To fulfill our duty to always do what is best for the patient, we must admit to ourselves and to each other when the status quo is causing harm. Likewise, parents also need to be empowered to advocate for change, because healthcare standards are unlikely to change *unless parents demand it*.

We implore those who write breastfeeding, jaundice, and hypoglycemia guidelines to *choose the safest and most conservative thresholds* and to err on the side of feeding to protect the infant brain. We implore them to stop glorifying one form of feeding while disparaging others. While breastfeeding should be protected and supported—and *absolutely* saves lives around the globe—so does properly prepared formula. The reality is that we need *both* to protect the health and futures of infants worldwide.

We believe that parents and babies are naturally equipped with the instincts they need for safe and successful feeding. Your instincts and your baby know that "fed is best." All everyone needs to do is listen.

ACKNOWLEDGMENTS

LYNNETTE HAFKEN

I dedicate this work to all the parents who have trusted me, at the most vulnerable time in their lives, with what is most precious in the world to them. You have *all* given your babies the very best start in life! I also dedicate this to the parents who have shared their painful stories; we are deeply grateful for your bravery and selflessness. Special thanks to my husband and soulmate, Dave Hafken, for being my partner in life; to my three beloved children, wonderful people who bring me infinite joy every day; Miranda Silvious, for being my Good Sister and a phenomenal mother to my nephew; my mother, Dr. Judith Terrill (née Devaney), for nurturing my mind with her passion for science; my father, Dr. Kenneth Schatten, for teaching me to speak truth to power; Alexis Hafken, for her loving presence in my family's life; Drs. Marianne Neifert, Erica Rupar, Sandra Cuzzi, Enrique Gomez, Nicole King, and Stephanie Perdue; Drs. Brooke Orosz and Ruth Anne Harpur; Sue Haddon, Cheri Wissman, Kavin Senapathy, Brean Schaffer, Kelli Arnette, and Katherine Morrison; to all the lactation professionals and mother–baby RNs who work so hard for babies and families every day; to Christie, one of the best and bravest people I know; to Jody, who "gets it" like no one else; and to La Leche League, for teaching me to listen to mothers, because they are the experts on their babies.

JODY SEGRAVE-DALY

Writing this book was one of the most challenging yet rewarding experiences of my thirty-two-year nursing career. It wouldn't have been possible without my husband, Steve, who afforded me the devotion of spending thousands of hours researching and writing for this book. His expertise as an obstetrician and gynecologist was available to me in many situations, and it was his unwavering support and love that enabled me to endure the constant Herculean battles I faced while publicly advocating for safe breastfeeding and perinatal mental health over the last seven years.

Thank you to my beloved sons, Josh, Dylan, and Matthew, who taught me to become a fierce mama bear and a staunch advocate for voiceless and vulnerable children. I am deeply grateful to my parents for teaching me to be brave and do the right thing no matter what, even if it means doing it alone.

I would like to thank Christie, my phenomenal partner, for exposing the current policies that promote exclusive breastfeeding through your relentless research, which indicates that hospitals worldwide must make immediate changes before implementing these policies, to protect newborns from complications caused by inadequate feeding. Despite others' attempts to silence you, you have made a tremendous impact on the globe by advocating for babies who need more milk to thrive.

The nurses and IBCLC colleagues I work with, especially Lynnette, give me hope that changes to promote safe breastfeeding are possible. To all of the parents who reached out to me with your infant feeding stories, you gave me the strength to continue on my most challenging days, knowing our work was helping countless families who were left confused and alone when their breastfeeding experience was traumatic. I will be eternally grateful to the many volunteers who kept our support group going while I was busy writing. Thank you for ensuring the most vulnerable parents are cared for daily.

Precious Landon Johnson, the angel who forever changed my nursing and lactation career, deserves my tribute. Based on what I read in his medical records, he didn't need to suffer or die because he did not consume enough milk while exclusively breastfeeding in the hospital. Landon's death made clear my professional, ethical, and moral responsibility and strengthened my resolve to advocate for newborns worldwide who lack adequate nutrition due to flawed breastfeeding policies.

CHRISTIE DEL CASTILLO-HEGYI

I want to thank my loving and supportive husband, Michael, whom I could not have done any of this without. I would love to thank my co-warriors and coauthors, Jody and Lynnette, who have volunteered thousands of hours and sacrificed so much to change the world for *all* moms, families, and babies. Thank you to Natalie Lakosil, our amazing book agent; Kristen Coghlan for all the beautiful artwork; Julia Bennett for helping us launch the Fed Is Best Foundation and the book's landing page; and Jennifer Achilles, MD, for helping us with our content. I want to thank our incredible BenBella editor-in-chief, Leah Wilson, who spent countless hours making this the best book possible. I want to thank James Fraleigh, our copy editor, and our production team at BenBella, as well as Kellie Doherty, our marketer. I want to thank Elizabeth Cumby, Diana Hegyi, Hugh Hegyi, and so many aunts and uncles in the Philippines for supporting me in this mission. I want to thank my mom, Beth, and my dad in heaven, Tante, for making my life and all the joy within it possible. I want to thank my brothers, Roehl, Carlo, Arnel, and Dennis, who taught me to be tough, so I can fight hard battles. I want to thank my smart and strong girls, Ella and Sage, for putting up with so many days when I had to write. Finally, I dedicate this work to Kai, who came into this world to right a wrong and to change it for the better.

ENDNOTES

The endnotes are available at the QR code below.

PHOTO CREDITS

Page 83 © Bricolage/Shutterstock

Page 89 © 2008 Charlotte Burns and Mary Rutherford, *Pediatrics*, published by the American Academy of Pediatrics

Pages 140, 212, 271, and 280 by Kristin Coghlan

Page 142 courtesy Alleigh Cooper

Page 148 © Beneda Miroslav/Shutterstock

Page 173 © SeventyFour/Shutterstock

Page 180 © phakimata - Can Stock Photo Inc.

Page 208 courtesy Rachel Boop

Page 224 courtesy Kristen Umunna

Page 252 courtesy Sandra Stephany Lozoya

Page 270 © Ground Picture/Shutterstock

Page 272 © 2020 Fiona Orr, Christina Hourigan, Cathrine Fowler, et al, *Maternal & Child Nutrition* published by John Wiley & Sons, Ltd.

Page 290 courtesy Abbie Fox

INDEX

nutrition
    caloric requirement of newborns,
        43–46
    with exclusive breastfeeding, 35–37,
        45–46
    in formula, 227, 231–233
    nutritional content of breast milk,
        209
    nutritional content of colostrum, 34,
        42–46
    nutritional requirements, 17–18 (*see
        also* safe and sufficient feeding)

O
obstetricians, 114
overfeeding, 41–42, 269–270, 281

P
paced feeding, 281
pacifier use, 67
parent education, 5, 5–14
    bias in, 119
    hospital discharge without, 123
    incomplete, 105–106, 145
    on lactation insufficiency, 74
    trusted information sources,
        116–119
partially hydrolyzed formula, 230, 233
PC–06, 12, 126
Pediatric Endocrine Society (PES), 87
pediatricians
    first visit to, 167–168
    on support team, 114–115
perception of insufficient milk (PIM),
    33
Perez-Escamilla, Rafael, 38
Philipp, Bobbi, 12, 13
phototherapy, 12, 98–99, 126
postpartum depression and anxiety,
    198–200
prelacteal feeding, 46, 50–55, 105
premature babies, 163–164
preparing to feed, 111–146

breastfeeding, 131–141
combo-feeding from the beginning,
    144–145
documenting feedings, 130
feeding plan, 112–113
formula feeding exclusively, 145–146
hospital/birth facility's policies,
    services, care, 119–127
monitoring newborn weight,
    127–130
signs of a well-fed newborn, 127
supplemental nursing systems,
    141–142
supplementing if necessary,
    142–144
support team, 113–116
trusted information sources,
    116–119
professionals, 291
    and breastfeeding complications,
        6, 7
    breastfeeding recommendations,
        3–4, 11–13, 28–32, 71
    ethical requirements for, 59
    lactation, 115–116
    questions to ask about feeding,
        119–127
    on support team, 113–116
    when to seek feeding evaluation
        from, 156–157, 156–157
    who offer formula, repercussions for,
        57–58
Promotion of Breastfeeding
    Intervention Trial (PROBIT), 42,
    63–66, 69, 175
pumped milk feeding, 207–222
    bottles for (*see* bottle feeding)
    breast pumps for, 132, 211–214
    direct latching vs., 207–209
    and drops in milk production,
        221–222
    feeding plans for, 112, 113
    mental health with, 220–221

ABOUT THE AUTHORS

Christie del Castillo-Hegyi, MD, is a board-certified emergency physician who studies newborn brain injury and developmental disabilities caused by insufficient feeding. She cofounded the Fed Is Best Foundation when her own first-born son was harmed by unsafe advice on exclusive breastfeeding from breastfeeding books and classes and from health professionals. When she learned that these complications were happening daily to infants across the globe as a result of things commonly taught to parents, she and Jody Segrave-Daly launched the Foundation to raise awareness among parents and health professionals. She has advocated for safer breastfeeding practices at the NIH, the USDA, and to members of Congress. Along with Segrave-Daly, she has met with the top officials of the World Health Organization breastfeeding guidelines program to discuss infants harmed by the exclusive breastfeeding policy. She has lectured at national medical conferences and published a case-report/review article on hypernatremic dehydration in exclusively breastfed newborns. She is a member of the Global Developmental Disabilities Research Collaborators and has coauthored papers documenting the rise in prevalence of multiple neurological and developmental disabilities among children worldwide.

Jody Segrave-Daly, RN, retired IBCLC, is a newborn nursery and newborn intensive care unit (NICU) nurse and is a staunch advocate for evidence-based feeding practices and perinatal mental health. Jody's entire thirty-year nursing career has been dedicated to caring for healthy and medically fragile babies in the nursery and NICU, and she has provided community-based infant-feeding support as a neonatal nurse and IBCLC for twelve years. She has comforted thousands of mothers all over the world who have contacted her for infant-feeding consultations, who believed it was rare to underproduce breast milk and often felt betrayed by their healthcare teams, their own bodies, and the social pressure that insisted "Breast Is Best" for every family. Jody is the Fed Is Best Foundation's clinical and education director, director of global outreach, and social media content developer. In addition to writing evidence-based educational resources, she has implemented change by debunking infant-feeding myths. Many of her resources have gone viral and have made a difference. She wrote the article "How to Breastfeed During the First 2 Weeks of Life" for the *New York Times Parenting Edition*.

Lynnette Hafken, MA, IBCLC, is a hospital and private practice lactation consultant, former La Leche League Leader, and advocate for family-centered lactation and infant-feeding support. She currently teaches a course for healthcare providers on safe and compassionate care for their breastfeeding patients. Lynnette's goal throughout her twenty-year vocation has been to help families breastfeed in a safe, enjoyable, and sustainable way, and in some cases to transition to infant formula while knowing their babies would thrive from being loved and fed. As the Foundation's director of support services, Lynnette applies her gift for listening to and connecting with parents to the advancement of the Fed Is Best vision for inclusive infant-feeding support.